Improving Quality and Reducing Cost with Electronic Health Records:

Case Studies from the
Nicholas E. Davies Awards

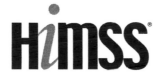

HIMSS Mission

To lead change in the healthcare information and management systems field through knowledge sharing, advocacy, collaboration, innovation, and community affiliations.

For more information about HIMSS, please visit www.himss.org.

Contents

Introduction 1
By Patricia Wise, RN, MSN, MA, FHIMSS

Section I
DAVIES ORGANIZATIONAL AWARD WINNERS

1995
Columbia-Presbyterian Medical Center 19
U.S. Department of Veterans Affairs 23
Intermountain Healthcare 27

1996
Brigham and Women's Hospital ** 31
Group Health Cooperative of Puget Sound ** 39

1997
Kaiser Permanente of Ohio 45
North Mississippi Health Services 49
Regenstrief Institute for Health Care 53

1998
Kaiser Permanente Northwest 57
Northwestern Memorial Hospital ** 61

1999
Kaiser Permanente Colorado Region 67
The Queen's Medical Center 71

2000
Harvard Vanguard Medical Associates 77
Veterans Affairs Puget Sound Health Care System 81

2001
Heritage Behavioral Health Center, Inc. 85
Ohio State University Health System 91
University of Illinois at Chicago Medical Center 97

2002
Maimonides Medical Center ** 101
Queens Health Network ** 109

_____

** Expanded profile provided

2003

Cincinnati Children's Hospital Medical Center 115

2004

Evanston Northwestern Healthcare 121

2005

Citizens Memorial Healthcare 127

Section II
DAVIES AMBULATORY CARE AWARD WINNERS

2003

Cooper Pediatrics 135

Evans Medical Group 139

Roswell Pediatric Center 143

2004

North Fulton Family Medicine 147

Old Harding Pediatric Associates 151

Pediatrics at the Basin 155

Riverpoint Pediatrics 159

2005

Southeast Texas Medical Associates, LLP 163

Sports Medicine & Orthopedic Specialists, PC 167

Wayne Obstetrics & Gynecology 171

Index 175

Introduction

Patricia Wise, RN, MSN, MA, FHIMSS
Colonel, USA Ret'd
Vice President, Health Information Systems
HIMSS

The HIMSS Nicholas E. Davies Award Program provides the nation's largest collection of first-hand accounts of the vision, leadership, technology and management required to achieve successful electronic health record (EHR)* implementation in large healthcare organizations and ambulatory practices. This book is a remarkable collection of "executive summaries" or profiles of award recipients' applications from both the organizational and ambulatory tracts of the Davies Program from the time period of 1995 through 2005.

Five of the earlier organizational winners are presented with expanded profiles. The Davies Program understands that the implementation of an EHR is not the goal but part of a continuum as information technology provides caregivers with tools to improve their quality and efficiency for their patients' wellbeing. Therefore, it was interesting to discover what these award-winning institutions accomplished in the years following a successful implementation.

The Davies Award Program, modeled after the Baldridge Award, was conceived by Computer-based Patient Record Institute (CPRI) in 1994 and launched a year later. Today, the Davies Award Program is proudly sponsored by HIMSS following the merger with CPRI in 2002. The program is named to honor the accomplishments and visions of Dr. Nicholas E. Davies, an Atlanta-based practicing physician who was tragically killed in a plane crash in 1991. At the time of his death, Dr. Davies was President-Elect of the American College of Physicians and a member of the Institute of Medicine (IOM) Committee on Improving the Patient Record. The report from this committee, released shortly after the death of Dr. Davies, called for the implementation of computer-based systems in hospitals to facilitate safety and quality in healthcare. The program is designed to nationally recognize, highlight, and share strategies and lessons learned from successful implementations.

More than a decade later, the Davies Program helps organizations and practices gain from the collective experiences of EHR implementations across the nation. Strategies and approaches are shared providing guidance and insight for healthcare organizations

---

* In this book, the terms electronic health record (EHR) and electronic medical record (EMR) are synonymous, although only the term EHR is used throughout.

preparing to invest substantial resources to more efficiently and effectively manage the care they provide. Additionally, the program seeks to document the value of EHRs for patients, clinicians and healthcare organizations and practices. Currently, there are three Davies tracts; Organizational for healthcare enterprises, Ambulatory for independent ambulatory primary care and specialty practices and Public Health.

Applicants for an Organizational Davies Award first submit a Threshold Application which addresses the content and scope of the EHR to be considered for the Davies Award, how the system integrates data from multiple sources, how and what types of decision support are provided, and evidence that the EHR is the primary source of clinical information for providers. The responses to the threshold criteria are reviewed and selected applicants are invited to submit a full application. The full applications are reviewed utilizing the Davies Framework to guide the assessment.

The Davies Framework for Evaluating Electronic Health Records presents a number of criteria which help applicants focus on key decisions, approaches and strategies of EHR implementation. Applicants are asked to produce evidence that these decisions and organizational strategies contributed to the success of the EHR implementation. The emphasis is on the implementation and the value derived from the system, not the choice of technology, design, or system platform. Site visits are conducted to ensure the veracity of the application and to gain additional insights into the organization. Ambulatory practice applications are also reviewed against a framework of criteria followed by a site visit.

The evaluation criteria contains four major sections; management, functionality, technology, and value. In the late 1990s organizations had difficulty quantifying the return on investment by traditional business calculations, so early Davies applicants were evaluated for the impact the system had on the organization. By 2002 the impact criterion became value-oriented with organizations and practices expected to address the return on investment. Readers will discover that the profiles presented follow the applications and provide strategies, decision points, and lessons learned in key areas.

LEADERSHIP LESSONS[1]

There are many clichés about leadership, most of them true. Leadership in healthcare does indeed start at the top, as in most industries. Solid executive leadership does make things happen. No Davies Award winner has achieved a successful EHR installation without the vision and support of their organization's top leaders, as well as supervisors and managers. Leadership is required to select appropriate vendors, plan the implementation, corral the support of physicians and staff, and navigate the inevitable rough patches that form during the dramatic transformations an EHR brings to institutions.

Support from the top is a prerequisite of good EHR installations and a strong indicator of good leadership. **Maimonides Medical Center** in Brooklyn found it was crucial to have "a strong CEO prepared for the expected difficulties, especially with the community-based physicians." In their award application Maimonides wrote, "When necessary, the CEO brought together the various constituencies in the organization to solve problems together."

Queens Health Network's CEO "has been tireless in his promotion of the system, endorsing it in public and private sessions throughout the organization and never ceasing to encourage the recalcitrant or reluctant to implement it."

The CEO of **Citizens Memorial Healthcare** visited his vendor's headquarters and participated as the keynote speaker at the launch of the EHR. He "expressed confidence in the success of the implementation" and the positive impact it would have on patient care, the hospital wrote in its Davies submission.

Boards of directors can play an equally important role. "The board of directors drove strategic planning, which focused on developing an organizational culture in which patient safety was the number one priority," wrote the authors of **Cincinnati Children's** submission. Having leadership declare automated patient records a strategic goal helps ensure a smoother transition to electronic records. **Evanston Northwestern Healthcare** "laid the foundation for success" by "making it the number one goal for the corporation for three years," according to its submission.

But leadership at the top is only part of the story. At **Queens Health Network** the medical director "insisted" on a system a physician could use easily and that had enhanced decision support functions. At **Evanston Northwestern** the authors of the Davies submission wrote: "The project had complete support from leadership: When people were needed for testing, their managers made them available for testing. When an emergency meeting was needed, people mobilized at once. Resources were made available for the extensive and compulsory training and for the floor and unit coverage needed while staff was away at training."

Planning for an EHR begins with committees and lots of them. The more input planners receive, the more buy-in they achieve from management and staff. If every department has a seat at the table, implementation will proceed more smoothly because hospitals can add functionality to the EHR based on staff input and customize training and educational materials for various users.

The EHR planning committees often have been assigned the task of creating the vision, goals, and strategic objectives for EHRs. At **Cincinnati Children's**, a group of leadership teams created a list of nine objectives, from optimizing patient safety to enhancing research productivity. **Evanston Northwestern** focused on just four goals: improved patient safety through elimination of illegible orders and medication errors, access to the right patient data, accurate information in the records, and simplifying consistent processes throughout the organization.

To make the project less about IT and more about clinical improvement, some institutions created committees to oversee EHR projects outside the IS departments. **Evanston Northwestern** formed a "Medical Informatics" department to lead the EHR effort as a "clinical project" and has members supporting new systems, overseeing upgrades and working with operations to adjust workflow throughout the enterprise. A Physicians Advisory Group also contributed guidance to the system's IT department.

Not all Davies winners followed that approach. **Citizens Memorial** created an IS Steering Committee—comprising technologists as well as directors of clinical services, finance, home care, and other relevant departments—to handle a needs assessment, to align organizational strategic objectives with IT strategies, and to produce a series of guiding principles. **Ohio State** used an IT team, in association with clinical and administrative personnel, to produce six goals for computerization of the medical records system.

Mixing up the committees with representatives from different departments makes sense when leading an organization through the EHR implementation. "Cross-functional teams, with representatives from frontline staff to corporate leadership, led the project as Heritage completely overhauled critical direct care and support service processes to take fullest advantage of the new technology," **Heritage Behavioral Health** personnel wrote in their submission.

These same teams, sometimes in combination with others working under the rubric of EHR planning, often helped conduct vendor selection. **Ohio State** had its two teams write a request for proposals to various vendors. They also assisted in the actual vendor selection—along with hundreds of employees who, at meetings, had a chance to voice their support or concerns with technology solutions provided by the three finalists.

Citizens Healthcare's IS Steering Committee led the vendor selection but involved 39 teams of employees "at each step," which created "strong consensus around the plan from the organization." The teams were asked to think big about what a perfect system might do to help them in their jobs.

Part of the vendor selection responsibility pivots on the important decision of whether to create custom applications in-house, to contract with multiple vendors, or to use, primarily, one vendor. **The University of Illinois at Chicago** considered custom clinical applications but decided, in the end, its competencies lie in care of the sick, not software development. **Maimonides**, on the other hand, discovered "no single supplier could meet its requirements or deliver a truly integrated solution." It decided to work with four vendors and, after the implementation, spun off a for-profit business with one of them.

Two other areas of leadership noted in Davies submissions are undertaking risk assessment and establishing a business case for EHR implementation. In assessing risk, leaders look at how and why an implementation might fail and create safeguards to ensure that cannot happen. Likewise, by offering a business case for an EHR—rather than using fallbacks such as "it's a good idea" or "it's the right thing to do"—executive and clinical leaders create a gauge by which they can judge their progress.

Citizens Memorial, for instance, assumed a positive return within five years based on several goals: to grow admissions; to increase revenue by adopting standardized protocols and recording accurate coding; to decrease transcription charges; to eliminate five positions; and to jettison expenses associated with paper records. At **Evanston Northwestern**, the steering committee built its financial case on increased accuracy in diagnoses and medication administration, fewer receivables and fewer employees in billing, and centralized scheduling.

It's not all about money for some Davies winners. A much different and less elaborate business case can be found in the **University of Illinois at Chicago's** submission. The authors say the project had "no specific financial objectives" but laid out three general goals: to reduce supply costs, achieve reimbursement benefits, and also achieve revenue enhancements." The Chicago submission points out the driving force behind the project was never about saving money, but rather "centralizing ambulatory clinics in the new Outpatient Care Center" and creating a "longitudinal, electronic health record that would be available virtually across the organization."

Project risk plays into leadership, too. The committees and executive councils acknowledge project risk in a variety of ways prior to an EHR implementation, and then plan as much as possible to mitigate those challenges. One of the greatest risk factors is staff buy-in—the fear that personnel will not adopt new standards or adapt to new ways of doing business. The other largest challenge arises from the potential downtime during implementation.

Cincinnati Children's believed user acceptance posed the greatest threat to its EHR project. To mitigate that concern, the institution created a design team staffed by physicians who received compensation to attend meetings and review design standards. Another team of nurses helped with the clinical documentation platform. The hospital hired a consulting firm to handle project management and embarked upon a public relations campaign 18 months before the first implementation, talking to internal groups as well as newspaper and television reporters. The hospital also carefully chose the first units for implementation based on the likelihood of success.

Citizens Memorial laid out eight areas of risk, nearly all of them associated with the possibility of staff rejection of the EHR. Techniques were adopted to checkmate each of the risks. For instance, the hospital system feared "known problem people" would resist change. It decided to solve that issue by identifying those people early and "make a positive effort to engage them in the process." Some end users may lack computer skills, the risk assessment concluded, but the institution would overcome that problem with training.

While undertaking its EHR, **Heritage Behavioral Health Center** grew concerned about lost productivity and staff resistance. To minimize disruptions, Heritage developed a training and certification program for staff and offered a technical help desk to assist users having problems with the new system. The institution also deployed a marketing team to promote the EHR and participate in pilot projects and to offer input on screen designs and process improvements. They "became vocal champions of the project."

Most inherent EHR implementation risks can be addressed through communication and education, and by maintaining an open environment. There is a consensus among Davies winners:

- Staff members must be kept up-to-date on a project's progress.
- Staff members must receive good training (an issue dealt with in greater detail in the implementation section below) and should be offered opportunities to learn in different modalities, from live presentations to online learning and written materials.
- Staff members must also have the opportunity to provide input and see that their best suggestions are incorporated into the project.

IMPLEMENTATION LESSONS[2]

Contained within the four sections of the evaluation criteria are the pearls of the Davies Award Program. Organizational and ambulatory winners describe in detailed first person accounts the steps and missteps along the path toward full EHR implementation.

Responding to the management criteria, organizations discuss their plans for transition from paper to electronic. Some organizations choose and implement systems quickly—the "big bang"—often using one or a few vendors to create interoperating systems that maximize the clinical benefits of healthcare information technology as rapidly as possible. Others plan a gradual implementation in order to ease the pains of transition from paper to electronic and give the organization a chance to learn from the mistakes and successes of each clinical department as the system is rolled out. Some organizations lay down the gauntlet and demand the physicians adapt to an electronic environment, or, at least, in one case, risk the right to refer patients to the hospital. Others use the carrot and stick approach, urging doctors to adapt by stressing the benefits, sometimes even relying on peer pressure to get reluctant clinicians to make the change.

One theme that is consistent throughout Davies winners is the need, once the decision is made to implement a clinical IT system, to devise an overarching strategic plan for the EHR. These plans generally result from meetings among planning teams, during which a series of sweeping objectives are presented. The planning teams often include members of the hospital administration, management staff, board members, and medical staff. Leadership from the CEO on down demonstrated tremendous commitment to going electronic across the continuum of care. Leadership teams were assembled, and while mistakes and misjudgments were occasionally made, a premium was always placed on orderly and effective communication of the organization's goals.

As part of a holistic planning process, many Davies winners conducted risk assessments and outlined approaches to mitigate the challenges they determined they were facing. **Cincinnati Children's Hospital Medical Center** thought their greatest risk management issue was the prospect that clinicians might not buy into the organizations' commitment to clinical IT. "Live planning sessions with a clinical unit that involved key managers and staff leaders from the patient care area were a good predictor of support that would be needed to ensure success at the time of the implementation and to sustain the project in that area."

Once the strategy for clinical IT is in place, the process of acquiring technologies that meet the institution's needs begins. Again, there are many paths to choose from, but Davies winners mainly have chosen among a best of breed approach, an integrated system, building a self-produced custom system, or buying off-the-shelf. They also had to decide whether to bring in consultants.

Perhaps the most important early decision organizations must make is whether to employ an integrated systems strategy or a "best of breed" approach. Integrated systems involve multiple clinical applications with a common database and uniform user interface, giving various modules a similar look and feel. Best-of-breed systems generally involve at least a primary if not solo vendor and are designed to excel in one or several applications. However, some important features may not be available at all, and the systems may require intensive training and support, impose complex system interfaces on users, or pose other problems.

After an institution decides what type of system it will acquire, it moves onto aquisition. This, obviously, is a key step in the process and one of the points along the path at which clinician buy-in can be doomed, along with the EHR project itself, if stakeholders are not closely involved.

The more recent Davies winners have enjoyed the luxury the earliest Davies award recipients clearly did not have: clinical information technologies that had already been road tested by their caregiver peers. This is one of the reasons why the most recent Davies winners owe a huge debt to EHR trailblazers such as **Intermountain Health Care** of Salt Lake City (Davies winner, 1995); Boston's **Brigham and Women's Hospital** (1996); Indianapolis-based **Regenstrief Institute for Health Care** (1997); and a host of other healthcare pioneers.

Project governance is a key aspect in the management of an EHR implementation. Careful, thoughtful oversight and engaged leadership are hallmarks of every Davies-winning implementation. Different organizations approached governance in various ways. Depending on the institution, EHR governance might fall under the aegis of one committee, or a combination of many project teams. Hospitals frequently had separate governing bodies overseeing implementation.

A critical step in the implementation process happens after the technology is in place; teaching end users to successfully navigate and utilize the technology and consistently supporting them as they gain EHR proficiency. In its award application, **Cincinnati Children's** refers to training as "communication, education, and support." Davies winners tried numerous training methods including **Maimonides Medical Center's** "just-in-time" training administered according to a specialty or department, using a physician-approved curriculum. Essentially the trainers focused on the "human aspect," finding the most comfortable way for end users to learn the technology. Another surprising tack that helped **Maimonides** convince physicians to adopt the new electronic technology was the decision to work training around the physician schedules, rather than trying to force doctors to work their schedules around training.

VALUE OR RETURN ON INVESTMENT (ROI) LESSONS[3]

Davies applications utilize the term "soft return on investment" for clinical variables promulgated by EHRs in such areas as patient safety, process improvement, and regulatory compliance. In their written applications, Davies Award winners offer detailed analysis in these categories, though they do not always include hard statistical data that proves their business cases.

It may be that many such factors are simply immeasurable. Unlike the many industrial companies that practice Six Sigma principles—a process improvement protocol requiring reams of data—healthcare providers face many challenges in quantifying every aspect of their practices. Although every treatment made by a physician or a nurse is chargeable, as lengthy medical bills attest, they are not always definable in terms of "hard" ROI or dollars seen on the bottom line.

Still, soft ROI carries just as much—and possibly more—importance to healthcare institutions, because many soft-return factors are transformative. Reducing errors in medication through decision support systems saves lives. Having access to a patient's entire healthcare history helps improve care. Aggregated data analysis assists in focusing providers on performance enhancements. EHR software offers a wealth of clinical data, and in that data can be found the seeds of improvement, change, challenge, and success.

The healthcare industry sees improving patient safety as a major imperative, especially as an Institute of Medicine study in 1999 revealed that as many as 98,000 Americans may be dying every year as a result of missed diagnoses, fatal drug interaction, and inappropriate treatment by physicians and nurses.

The Joint Commission on Accreditation of Healthcare Organizations (JCAHO) has made improving patient safety one of seven initiatives for the coming year. Davies winners invariably cite patient safety as one of the prerogatives of implementing an EHR in their hospitals.

Evanston Northwestern Healthcare writes that "the vision of a paperless system" promised to "improve patient safety by eliminating problems associated with illegible orders and medication orders." Under its "mission and vision" section, **The Ohio State University Health System** cited its desire to "maximize the quality of patient care" as its number one goal for having an EHR. **Cincinnati Children's Hospital Medical Center** saw "optimizing patient safety" as the first of nine strategic objectives. **Citizens Memorial Healthcare**, a rural provider, saw patient safety as "eliminating handwriting/transcription errors by requiring completeness of orders through clinical decision support, and by providing access to clinical information and a patient medical history."

In fact, simple things such as replacing the poor handwriting of harried physicians move healthcare providers toward more accurate treatment of patients while reducing the time staff and pharmacists devote to dealing with drug interactions or prescribing issues. EHR software embedded with decision support alerts physicians, nurses, and other staff to the potential for prescription problems while helping them automatically calculate dosages based on patient characteristics.

The Davies Award winners cite a number of patient safety improvements in several areas in addition to improving prescription practices. Here is a glimpse at some of the data submitted in their award proposals:

Maimonides Medical Center, a 705-bed hospital, saw problem medication orders drop by 58 percent and medication discrepancies by 55 percent in 2001 after its EHR implementation. That same year, the decision support feature identified 164,250 alerts, resulting in 82,125 prescription changes. The provider's EHR addressed "high alert medications," confusing look-alike and sound-alike drug names, as well as patients with similar names that could potentially cause the pharmacy confusion.

Queens Health Network experienced a 50 percent decrease in pharmacist interventions in medication orders in ambulatory care because of improved legibility, system alerts, and increased completeness of prescriptions. Due to point-of-care availability of real-time patient information, the hospital network has seen reduced numbers of admissions resulting from warfarin toxicity, a common problem when drug dosages are wrong.

Online medication charting saw errors in transcription drop to zero for departments in which EHRs were in full use at **Ohio State University Health System**. In areas where the EHR had not been implemented, transcription errors ran as high as 26 percent in its system. Other healthcare providers also saw transcription errors drop to zero.

Evanston Healthcare found that new procedures regarding a medication could be introduced in just hours. Problems with Dilaudid, for example, brought about different recommended doses in patients. The hospital changed 32 order sets and 22 preference lists in 3 hours. In one week, a physician-led pathway team designed a risk-assessment tool for blood clots in legs, now used throughout the hospital. The healthcare provider also found that omitted administration of medications decreased 22 percent, from a total of 18 to 14 a month.

Cincinnati Children's, a 324-bed hospital, found medication errors dropped by 50 percent and mislabeled laboratory specimens, another area of concern, decreased to nearly zero. Care orders for common diagnoses such as asthmaticus, bronchiolitis, and gastroenteritis often had followed no set guidelines previously, but these, too were improved. Using evidence-based guidelines found in the EHR, the hospital showed a 20 percent improvement in the consistency of care for bronchiolitis, for example.

Summarizing all the process improvements that come with an EHR implementation is difficult. Many healthcare providers use several pages in their applications simply describing how their EHRs encouraged them to change communication and workflow to reflect their newfound ability to access patient records from multiple locations.

A common user interface is one process improvement that allows hospital personnel to navigate user-friendly screens to locate patient data, in stark contrast to the hodgepodge of software systems and interfaces many hospitals employed in the past. By using consistent electronic data sets for every patient—again, a novelty because paper medical charts changed over time, creating difficulties when attempting to compare information—healthcare providers now can standardize both data and care.

Other improvements come with eliminating duplicate records and from electronic charting and discharge, electronic signatures, patient check-in, and access to referring physician information. The physician inbox of many software systems can display documents to sign and review, phone messages, and consult orders. In the past, this all required a large stack of folders, pink callback slips, and other paper forms. In addition, instructions to nurses tend to be clearer and more precise with an EHR. Duplicate testing dropped dramatically. At **Maimonides**, ancillary tests decreased by 48.9 percent, urinalysis by 41.6 percent, microbiology by 40.6 percent, and hematology by 6 percent.

The software recognizes most patients. At **Citizens Memorial,** the software has records on 92 percent of patients the institution sees. At Queens, 100 percent of the patients have electronic records. Previously, in the paper medical chart environment, Queens' staff could only find charts for 70 percent of patients.

Warnings, or alerts, improve care. At **Ohio State**, a five-hospital system, the EHR's alerts and flags cue physicians to orders requiring co-signatures, abnormally high or low results, changes in a patient's location, and orders to ancillary departments such as radiology, laboratory, pharmacy, dietary, and respiratory therapy.

At **Citizen's Memorial** and at other providers, physicians now have the option of entering orders at hospitals or long-term care facilities, or even remotely, and many choose to do so: "Orders are compared in real-time with rules and standards designed to reduce errors and improve quality of care, including medication interactions, allergy checking, presentation of pertinent results, and order-specific rules."

The time to deliver medications dropped dramatically. At **Maimonides,** it fell by 68 percent, from 276 minutes on average to 88 minutes. **Ohio State** saw the time it took to obtain medications from the pharmacy drop from 3 hours and 14 minutes to 1 hour and 22 minutes.

The presence of EHRs greatly enhances communication among providers and patients. Something as simple as legible documentation, rather than physician scrawl, helps pharmacists offer the right medications at the right dosages. Something as complex as decision support reminds doctors to suggest patients get Pap smears, mammograms, blood-pressure checks, vaccinations, and so forth. Communications can make a world of difference in a large provider environment.

The Davies' award winners cite many examples of increased communications:

• **Citizens Memorial** physicians send a "Message to Nursing" with specific instructions or information on a patient. The hospital system's EHR is available from any of its care locations and any hospital department, eliminating the need for transport of documents. The physician desktop also alerts staff of prescription refill requests and laboratory results.

• **Queens Health Network's** EHR allows for sharing of documentation by all staff. The nursing staff's "documentation of vital signs, immunizations, fingerstick glucose testing, PPDs, etc., are available online at all times across the continuum of care," states Queens' submission. The process "helps eliminate duplication of effort, and, more importantly, encourages users to read what other caregivers have documented."

• **Cincinnati Children's** uses different font color (blue) to inform nursing they have a new order; it changes to black when the order is completed. Electronic order entry involving portable x-rays can be combined with pager notification to alert, for example, the radiology department of the need for its services.

• **Maimonides'** submission notes that laboratory and radiology results "are distributed electronically within 12 to 48 hours to a nursing pool where results are screened." Abnormal results go to the physician of record. Traditionally, that process took a week and the chance that abnormal results would be missed was much higher.

Hospitals are required to document their care to several important regulatory bodies and to their own oversight committees. They must also abide by new federal guidelines providing for patient privacy. The EHR software assists greatly in hospitals reaching for full compliance with a host of regulatory issues that will, in fact, lead to greater patient safety and better care.

The ability of physicians and nurses to document every patient encounter in the EHR, to view a patient's entire history in a consistent format, and to see best-practice treatment protocols helps enormously in complying with the myriad of healthcare regulations.

An additional point is worth making. By employing passwords and other security protocols that offer differing levels of failsafe user clearance, computerized health records can effectively restrict access to patients' confidential records. This makes complying with the Health Insurance Portability and Accountability Act of 1996 (HIPAA) that much easier. Later Davies winners often cited compliance with HIPAA as one of the chief advantages of their EHR deployments.

But HIPAA is not the only law providers need to abide. Those protocols promulgated by JCAHO, the Centers for Medicare and Medicaid (CMS), state agencies, and others that have oversight of hospitals and clinics also must be observed. Again, the data-crunching capabilities and alert systems inherent in EHR software help nurses and doctors comply with national and institution-based protocols.

Few award winners outlined in as great a detail as **Ohio State University Health System** the EHR's influence on regulatory compliance. The hospital found the EHR:

• Advanced full compliance with institutional policies and bylaws regarding do-not-resuscitate orders and restraint orders.

• Required staff to get a signature on an informed consent form from all patients undergoing chemotherapy.

• Allowed staff the ability to run daily reports for the Ohio State Pharmacy Board to exhibit compliance with a state directive that requires physicians to confirm their identities before administering controlled substances to patients. The hospital generates daily reports on quality initiatives for the Ohio Department of Health.

• Helped Ohio State comply with JCAHO and CMS mandates requiring allergy assessments and diagnosis upon admission. The EHR offers electronic discharge instructions by use of ICD-9 codes for primary admission diagnosis and discharge diagnosis. It also prompts certain questions to help charge entry clerks determine Medicare eligibility. The hospital's compliance is at 100 percent for co-signatures on all verbal orders.

Other award winners cite similar compliance advantages:

• **Cincinnati Children's** saw orders permanently unsigned by physicians drop from 40 percent to around 10 percent and witnessed a corresponding drop in verbal orders. Patient documentation was not previously performed in a timely manner and verbal orders for controlled substances were commonplace. With an EHR in place, the hospital saw a 24 percent reduction in verbal orders for controlled substances. Compliance with pain assessment protocols also jumped substantially.

• At **Queens Health,** completion of JCAHO-mandated summary lists—a required log of patient diagnoses, significant invasive and operative procedures, allergies and adverse drug reactions, and medications taken by patients—rose from 3.7 percent in a paper environment to 100 percent during a 6-month EHR conversion period.

• **Maimonides Medical** calls "aggregated data and information" a "very powerful" application. The hospital uses reports in the OB/GYN to improve performance and submits results to the state's Department of Health–Statewide Planning and Research Cooperative System, as mandated.

The definition of hard return on investment on EHRs involves two measurements: quantifiable returns that can be demonstrated in financial terms and process improvements that would suggest cost savings that may fit an identifiable—or measurable—metric. Physicians and nurses do not always measure their work with the kind of metrics available in other industries. Providers simply have not had the tools to conduct a thorough vetting of hard RIO. But with more sophisticated electronic systems now available to healthcare, the ROI equation is changing. These systems facilitate hard ROI data capture using more comprehensive methodologies.

In general, hard ROI from EHR installations can be grouped into three major categories: patient flow; materials and staffing reductions; and billing improvements. Some increases are astonishing; others show marginal—if still important—savings, or higher reimbursements.

Evidence of hard ROI is much richer in ambulatory care settings, perhaps because the data involves a smaller number of physicians and patients, and smaller, less diffuse budgets. Therefore, running the numbers and getting a feel for cost savings, patient flow, and billing yields a richer palette of statistics than is evident in larger hospitals and practices.

Only a handful of institutions looked at data that suggested an EHR installation could generate greater patient volumes, thereby increasing revenues and profitability. But there is anecdotal evidence that EHRs help healthcare providers move patients more efficiently through the care continuum. In fact, inpatient stays are generally shorter, and patients receive better care, on average, with an EHR in place. Hard data is, frankly, slender on this issue but several Davies winners report the following:

- **Citizens Memorial** saw net patient revenues increase 23 percent after the EHR implementation. It believes the EHR has had a positive impact on patient volume.
- Patient visits to **Maimonides'** emergency department increased from 57,795 in 1996 to 77,118 in 2002. Meanwhile, the average length of stay plummeted from 7.26 days in 1995 to 5.05 days in 2001, one full day less than the New York City average.
- **Ohio State's** data revealed a decline in the length of inpatient stays in a majority of services it offers, from transplant surgery to neurology.

Because EHRs reduce the need for paper, transcribers, and space for medical records, their introduction can reap immediate financial rewards. However, it is notable that a reduction in staff may not always occur, because employees who once performed data entry, for example, might be deployed in new areas. That kind of employee shifting, common at hospitals, alleviates the need to hire new employees.

Radiology is another area in which resources have been dramatically reallocated. Paper and non-digital film requires labor to organize, chart, file, and find, but computers perform the same tasks in seconds, not minutes or hours. Thus, digital radiology has been a key source of savings in many institutions.

Here are more examples of effective, EHR-inspired resource shifting:

- **Evanston Northwestern** increased volume with its EHR equivalent to eliminating 65 full-time employees throughout the corporation, or $4 million. The hospital reduced personnel in the emergency department, medical records and billing, as well as decreased overtime and temporary employee expenses. The total for all staff-related reductions equals $7.78 million. By eliminating forms, a scheduling system and dictation, the hospital saved another $1.94 million.

- Implementation of PACS and voice recognition systems, along with a radiology information system, saved $10.5 million at **Maimonides** over five years by eliminatin film, transcription, film jackets, and some hardware and software maintenance.
- **Heritage Behavioral Health** saved $473,859 over three years, in the following areas: $211,000 for transcription and documentation; $146,000 for chart audit paybacks; and $117,000 for back-office staffing reductions.
- **The University of Illinois at Chicago** reallocated $1.2 million of nurse time from manual documentation tasks to direct delivery of patient care. Charge nurses spent 2.75 hours less per week on medication administration, while caregiver nurses reported an hour less per week on this task after EHR implementation. Another $172,800 was saved in the health information department after chart assemblers increased their productivity as a result of online results and order access.
- **Queens Health Network** employed PACS and voice recognition systems, saving $993,000 per year at one of its hospitals, Elmhurst Hospital. Savings accrued from reductions in film and supplies; file-room space; personnel services for scheduling, filing, making appointments, and relaying results; and length of stay reductions also improved throughput. The hospital dropped five full-time positions and eliminated phone calls to obtain results. The radiology department at one Queens hospital saved another $164,000 in transcription costs, while its other hospital saved $206,200 in related expenses.
- At **Ohio State**, the implementation of PACS had equally impressive results, reducing film costs by $1.3 million annually. The hospital system also saved $70,000 collectively on paper, nursing time, and wasted medications, the last which resulted from a 50 percent reduction in medication errors and the complete elimination of transcription errors.

Clearly, having an EHR system clarifies the often-messy world of billing. Capturing charges is easier and is in real-time, so submissions to insurers can be completed digitally and within hours of treatment, rather than days. Studies show as much as 50 percent of care in some hospitals never gets submitted for reimbursement. The EHR function helps providers keep track of treatment and assists in coding for accurate billing. Davies Award winners cite billing improvements, through more complete bills and better collection, as hard ROI that eventually pays for the software. Here are a few examples:

- **Evanston Northwestern** saw a $2.5 million increase in revenue after solidly linking charge capture directly with orders. Improved coding edits and better emergency department charge capture added another $134,000, and flexible editing of claims contributed $48,000. A cumulative revenue increase of $2.68 million resulted from EHR use, and co-pay collection rates increased from 21 to 50 percent.
- At **Queens Health Network**, the claims denial rate decreased in one managed-care contract from 35 percent in the first quarter of 2001 to 21 percent in the first quarter 2002; another large facility Queens owns experienced a denial drop from 43 percent to 26 percent. Elmhurst, a Queens Health hospital, saw an increase in revenues from radiology of $306,000 during the first year of the EHR.

- **Heritage Behavioral Health,** an organization with several outreach programs, repaid $9,477 in 1994 to payors for non-compliant documentation or ineligible services. The figure in 2001, after the EHR implementation, was $774. The system saved another $39,000 on data entry in billing through staff reductions.
- **Citizens Memorial** experienced a decrease in accounts receivable for its physicians from more than 80 days to fewer than 50 days, by centralizing billing, charging functions, and consolidating the databases of 16 clinics. Automatic charge capture increased revenue $34 per patient. Claim denials have been reduced.
- **Ohio State** improved cash flow by allowing expedited payor payments to patient accounting systems. It electronically sends accounts to vendors for immediate follow-up and collection after conducting front-end edits to meet payor requirements.
- **Maimonides** watched as profits rose from $761,000 in 1996, before the EHR, to $6.1 million in 2001 after implementation, much of it a result of improved bill collection. The hospital attributes one-fourth of that revenue increase to the EHR and estimates it has enjoyed a 9.4 percent return on investment annually. Research by the hospital suggests that it has had a 4.84-year payback on its $43.8 million investment.

A SALUTE TO THE PIONEERS

The first Davies Awards were presented in 1995 to three institutions, **Intermountain Health Care** of Salt Lake City; the **Veterans Health Administration (VHA)** of Washington, DC; and **Columbia Presbyterian Medical Center** of New York. It is worth noting that one of those winners, Intermountain Health, observed in its submission that pioneers are "those having arrows in their backs." The vital contributions of those early award winners should not be overlooked.

The VHA's Decentralized Hospital Computer Program (DHCP) is the forerunner of today's VistA EHR, which serves as the foundation of a free EHR program being distributed by the federal government to small hospitals and practices. The program began in 1979 as an initiative launched by a small group of VA hospitals. As the feasibility of nascent EHRs became apparent, the agency began to perform cost-benefit analyses and feasibility studies and, finally, to fund the project. By 1982, the agency decided to take a decentralized approach to hospital IS, and DHCP was born. By the time of its 1995 Davies application, the program was the base information system for the entire Veterans Health Administration network, supporting 171 medical centers, 450 outpatient clinics, and 131 nursing homes.

The contributions of Intermountain Health Care also deserve special mention. The Utah institution's journey into clinical IT began four decades ago when what was then LDS Hospital began applying computer technologies to medical care. Those early homegrown experiments resulted in the creation of a system known as Health Evaluation through Logical Processing (HELP).

"While its creation was remarkable," the Intermountain submission's authors note, "the truly impressive feat was the acceptance it received from caregivers." In some ways, Intermountain Health may have dished up the prototype for all future EHR installations, both because of its early failures and the way they were overcome. The organization admits that its initial "pioneering phase" was "long on vision, but short on classic systems planning, such as governance, strategy, benchmarking, justification, etc."

But leadership evolved, and the system generated such promising results—and favorable local press coverage—that by 1987 it had secured the solid backing of Intermountain's board of directors. The board opted to continue funding the system, then known as IHCNet. "It has always been incumbent on information systems leadership to facilitate that commitment and remain flexible in light of evolving strategic priorities," IHC's authors write.

I would be remiss not to mention, finally, the pioneering efforts of **Brigham and Women's Hospital** (Davies winner, 1996), Boston's 712-bed academic medical center. Brigham and Women's pioneers, including über-CIO John Glaser, chose as their mandate "to build new clinical information systems that would change the computer's role in the healthcare process." It can be said that the institution proceeded a considerable distance by 1996 toward realizing its goal that "the computer would become an active partner in promoting optimal quality of care, reducing adverse events and reducing costs." The fact that it was successful, the organization's authors state, was due to several key factors: strong support for IT from the organization; "prescient" technical design decisions; a software design strategy that put the clinician first; intensive groundwork by the IS crew to prepare the institution for a major cultural shift; and quick responsiveness to user feedback. It might have added a sophisticated governance structure based on Brigham's philosophy that clinical IT requires individuals with significant knowledge of both IT and clinical practices.

ACKNOWLEDGMENTS

The profiles in this book are presented in the past tense and represent a point-in-time look and review of the EHR systems; the time when the organizations and practices were applying for the Davies Award. These profiles were developed based on their application, distilling as much as possible of the essence of their efforts, decisions and strategies. For more information on the Davies Program and to read the full applications go to www.HIMSS.org/davies.

The work of the Davies Program was first accomplished by CPRI volunteers and now by HIMSS volunteers who collectively have donated thousands of hours over the years to guarantee the success of this endeavor. They developed and periodically updated the criteria, reviewed threshold and full applications, participated in rousing committee debates and traveled throughout the country on site visits. HIMSS and the healthcare industry thank you. This outstanding program flourishes thanks to your efforts!

HIMSS would like to thank the five individuals who made it possible for us to provide additional information on their organizations' use of EHRs in the years following their Davies Awards: Diane M. Carr, formerly with Queens Health Network and now Deputy Executive Director, Operations, North Bronx Healthcare Network; Ted Eytan, MD, Medical Director, Health Informatics & Web Services, Group Health Cooperative; Maxine Fielding, Senior Director Clinical Systems, MIS Department, Maimonides Medical Center; Jonathan Teich, MD, PhD, Assistant Professor of Medicine, Harvard University Department of Emergency Medicine, Brigham & Women's Hospital; and

Timothy R. Zolph, Vice President of Information Services and Chief Information Officer, Northwestern Memorial Hospital.

REFERENCES

1. A Desire for Change: Strong Leadership Required in the EMR-EHR Revolution. White Paper. Chicago: HIMSS; 2006. Available at
   www.himss.org/ASP/davies_whitepapers.asp.

2. Making IT Happen: Strategies for Implementing the EMR-EHR. White Paper. Chicago: HIMSS; 2006. Available at
   www.himss.org/ASP/davies_whitepapers.asp.

3. The ROI of EMR-EHR: Productivity Soars, Hospitals Save Time and Yes, Money. Chicago: HIMSS; 2006. Available at
   www.himss.org/ASP/davies_whitepapers.asp.

SECTION I

DAVIES ORGANIZATIONAL AWARD WINNERS

1995 DAVIES ORGANIZATIONAL AWARD WINNER
COLUMBIA-PRESBYTERIAN MEDICAL CENTER

ABOUT THE ORGANIZATION

Columbia-Presbyterian Medical Center (CPMC) in New York City, New York, is one of the largest healthcare providers in the United States. At the time of the Davies Award, the main hospital had 1,190 beds, 55,000 admissions, 13,000 emergency visits, and 650,000 outpatient visits annually. The health sciences campus employed more than 6,000 people who worked in 13 buildings. CPMC also supported a community hospital of 300 beds, clinics and physician offices at separate locations, and a data center several miles away.

MANAGEMENT

CPMC leaders made a substantial investment in a computer-based patient record through its clinical information system (CIS). The sheer size of the organization provided a significant challenge to the vision and plans. The CPMC CIS was organized as a central hub that enabled clinical systems on disparate platforms to share patient data. System design was based on three guiding principles:

1. Patient data was a shared resource; it was necessary to construct a global view of a patient's care over time by integrating disparate information sources.
2. Patient data must be standardized to be shared.
3. Patient data must be monitored actively, not just passively stored.

The CIS model was developed to represent the events involving a patient in the healthcare setting—an inpatient admission, a clinic visit, or a physician office visit. The collection of events constituted a longitudinal record of care. The approach taken was a generic data model that provided a template for clinical events. The real content of each event was provided by one or more detail items. Every item was defined as a concept in the Medical Entities Dictionary (MED). The MED contained more than 40,000 terms related to admission, discharge, laboratory, pharmacy, cardiology, radiology, patient problems, and diseases.

The CPMC network and much of the infrastructure was built as part of the integrated advanced information management system (IAIMS), of which the CIS was just one component. The IAIMS, funded by the National Library of Medicine, also provided information to support scholarly, administrative, clinical research, and basic science activities.

By 1995, CIS workstations were located throughout the hospital, in clinical departments, physician offices, house staff areas, and other locations. Users also could dial in from home. The network extended to almost all areas of the organization.

FUNCTIONALITY

Creation of the CIS required integration efforts at two levels. The first was to integrate disparate hardware platforms by means of the network. The second involved integrating applications written by different vendors using different software platforms.

Network integration was achieved first by establishing connectivity to the token ring or Ethernet. Integration of different clinical software was achieved through use of the Health Level Seven (HL7) protocol for data exchange. As new systems were purchased, CPMC required vendors to provide two HL7 interfaces: one to serve as a transaction log of critical events, and the other to receive information from the central hub.

It was crucial for the CIS to be able to incorporate new technology to maximize the life span of the system and to achieve the best price-to-performance ratio for equipment. First, the client/server paradigm facilitated greater independence of front-end systems from back-end systems. In addition, the CIS architecture was based on separate components—database, dictionary, and event monitor—that could be enhanced independently.

The CIS standard data exchange interfaces facilitated communication with external parties. The client/server paradigm allowed information services to be performed separately by outside groups, which could provide the service more cost effectively. For example, diagnostic information from a commercial laboratory like MEDPATH was easily incorporated into the CIS. Information services were readily available to affiliated hospitals and physician offices.

TECHNOLOGY

The CIS central hub included a series of concentric layers. The message-handling layer received requests from client applications on the network to either store or retrieve data. Requests were composed using a standard message syntax, which enabled applications on a variety of platforms to communicate with CIS. Messages were queued, verified, logged, and passed to the inner layers of the hub.

The transition layer mapped data elements being stored in the system into a standard representation. Data to be stored in the clinical repository was defined in MED. The MED controlled the use of data elements by defining how variants mapped onto a single identifier denoted a unique concept.

Within the hub, the routing layer copied certain messages and sent them to target systems. The routing function was driven by tables indicating which messages should be copied, based on criteria such as the patient identifier, the location of a patient, and the type of message.

The monitoring layer triggered logic that evaluated the patient record by specific criteria. This review process was carried out by the Event Monitor program, which used a set of rules called Medical Logic Modules (MLMs) written in a high-level language. MLMs could provide alerts, management critiques, therapy suggestions, diagnosis scores, and screening for research studies.

In the access layer, messages were verified and interpreted, and data was stored in the clinical repository or retrieved.

Information needs varied widely throughout CPMC. Most groups could not wait for a central information service to select and purchase software or develop custom applications. As a result, the CIS allowed various software systems to run on different hardware platforms. This highly heterogeneous information environment was well supported by a sophisticated wide area network (WAN) that permitted front-end workstations to access a large number of back-end information services.

A variety of protocols coexisted on the network and collectively contributed to the client/server paradigm. The CPMC network featured more than 60 physical token rings, dozens of Ethernet segments, and a wide variety of hosts: three IBM 3090s, 45 minicomputers, 42 Novell servers, six PC local area network (LAN) servers, 20 IBM RS6000s, and a few operating system 2 (OS/2) LAN servers. The network supported 3,200 devices, including IBM PC workstations, Macintosh, X-stations, dumb terminals, terminal servers, and controllers. Most workstations ran in a disk operating system (DOS), with a simple menu interface that enabled access to a variety of applications. A few workstations ran MS Windows, and operating systems such as OS/2 and UNIX.

For system security and confidentiality, users had to be authorized to log on to the machine where an application was located and sometimes pass through additional security imposed by the application itself. All access to patient data was recorded in an audit trail. This data was reviewed regularly; violators were prosecuted. User sessions were subject to time outs to reduce the possibility of unauthorized use.

The integrity of clinical data was assured through the centralization of information services. When an application sent data to the central hub, the HL7 message was subject to validation checks: the message must have the correct syntax and contain all required elements; all data items must be defined in the dictionary to be translated into MED codes; the patient identifier must exist; and the patient's name must match within a certain tolerance level.

Database backups were performed nightly. The data was physically distributed over numerous storage devices, reducing the chances of large-scale data loss. These pieces could be recovered independently, reducing downtime.

The clinical repository and event monitor both resided on a single IBM mainframe. While the mainframe provided a robust platform, system failures were a concern. In the rare event of central processing unit (CPU) or system difficulties, the CIS could run on a second mainframe. Backups were made of the disk contents. Disk management software that greatly increased redundancy was acquired. Redundant physical paths in the network lessened the possibility of long outages when cables were severed or routers failed.

VALUE

The goal of the CPMC CIS was 24-hour availability, seven days a week. By 1995, planned downtime amounted to approximately one hour per month. Average response time for the CIS was 0.6 seconds during non-peak time, and 0.9 seconds during peak hours.

System data integrity, accuracy, and completeness were monitored monthly for reporting to internal quality assurance. Other measures included a reduction in average transmission time of lab results to two seconds, and electrocardiogram (EKG) reports, 24 hours from dictation to central storage.

CPMC leaders identified the greatest strength of the CIS architecture as "its ability to adapt to change; new applications could be added with relative ease and the components of the CIS itself could be replaced as new technology became available."

Indeed, the system was, and remains, under constant change. The network was extended, new servers and workstations were added, and new clinical applications were made available. The modular, distributed nature of the CPMC CIS and the use of standard interfaces and protocols greatly facilitated the continuing evolution of the system, with minimal impact on users.

1995 DAVIES ORGANIZATIONAL AWARD WINNER
U.S. DEPARTMENT OF VETERANS AFFAIRS

ABOUT THE ORGANIZATION

At the time it won the Davies Award in 1995, the U.S. Department of Veterans Affairs' Veterans Health Administration (VHA) met the healthcare needs of 2.6 million veterans through 171 medical centers, 450 outpatient clinics, 131 nursing homes, and 35 domicilaries. Veterans received 1.1 million inpatient episodes of care, 24 million outpatient visits, 50 million prescriptions, 250 million laboratory tests, and 1.3 million dental services in fiscal year 1993.

All of these services were supported through the VHA's Decentralized Hospital Computer Program (DHCP), a comprehensive and portable system covering medical management, fiscal, and clinical functions. Introduced in 1982, DHCP was considered by many to be an early computerized patient record (EHR) system. Each Veterans Affairs medical center (VAMC) could select from more than 60 integrated DHCP applications to build a flexible information system that supported its particular environment and mix of services.

MANAGEMENT

As part of its mission to provide high-quality healthcare for U.S. veterans, the VHA established the long-term goal of developing an EHR, which would build on the DHCP foundation. The EHR's goals were to enable the sharing and exchange of data, first throughout the VHA, then with other government organizations sharing a responsibility for federal healthcare, and eventually with private-sector organizations as standards-based open systems became achievable on an industry-wide level.

VHA took a modular, incremental approach to the EHR, giving clinicians data and functionality that were immediately useful while laying the foundation of a comprehensive patient information environment. To achieve this approach, VHA was guided by DHCP's principle: "Develop applications which are device and platform independent, and which permit the evolution and substitution of technologies within the constraints of budget limitations with a minimal impact on the application code, the system, and the users."

The EHR was expected to organize all relevant data on a patient in a way that directly supported clinical activity and indirectly fed management and administrative systems. These goals required the VHA to meet a number of major challenges, including migrating from a department-centered architecture to one that adequately supported both departmental and patient-centered functionality, and incrementally increased the scope of data contained in the system to respond to major changes in the VHA environment, such as primary care initiatives and healthcare reform.

The EHR's strategic objectives were as follows:
- Maximize value of the automated clinical information system (ACIS) across organizational lines.
- Incorporate the patient as a participant in the information system.
- Make comprehensive patient data available when and where it is needed.
- Implement an ACIS that is accepted and used by care providers.
- Treat end users as customers.
- Integrate ACIS and EHR as functional parts of the VHA organization.

VHA leadership appointed an Information Resources Advisory Council (IRAC) to recommend priorities in the development of applications; recommend, establish, and monitor the work of specific application requirements groups (ARGs); and monitor the appropriateness of implemented and planned information technology, among other responsibilities. Governance also included a clinical ARG, management ARG, information technology ARG, expert panels, and the medical information resources management office.

System security and patient confidentiality were assured through the VA Kernel software security module, which controlled user access to the system, the menus and options a user could gain access to, and the files and fields of data particular users were allowed to modify.

No major EHR acquisition was made because vendor and platform independence was a major objective. The 12-year (1983 to 1994) life cycle cost for DHCP was $1.2 billion. By 1994, expenditures for automation nationwide in the VHA had reached $321 million.

Application distribution was a mix of mandated and optional applications. Local implementation at the medical centers first focused on automation of existing processes, such as patient registration or operation of a clinical laboratory. Each application was assigned an automatic data processing application coordinator (ADPAC) to be the local expert on content and operation, but no additional staffing was provided due to the expected efficiencies. Training and education of VHA staff in the use of clinical record software was organized and supported by Regional Medical Education Centers and the Office of Academic Affairs.

FUNCTIONALITY

Definition of user information needs occurred through the ARG/expert panel structure. However, given the size of VHA, the organization experienced a significant challenge in obtaining adequate field input despite a very well defined needs-identification structure. Leadership implemented a new request processing system to address the challenge.

Expansion of the DHCP's clinical functionality for the EHR included the following:
- **Order entry and results reporting:** A new graphical user interface (GUI) provided clinicians with an easy-to-use, intuitive method of entering orders, and accessing and updating electronic charts.

- **Problem list:** List functionality was expanded in order to serve as a point of integration for the automated patient record for functions from billing to association of interventions and outcomes.
- **Discharge summary:** Both the administrative and clinical aspects of the summary were enhanced to support the capture, storage, and viewing of discharge summary data.
- **Health summary:** This summary gave clinicians the ability to browse through patient data interactively or generate a printed report.
- **Patient data exchange:** This function allowed a provider at one VAMC to request health summaries on patients from other VAMC.
- **Patient care encounter (PCE):** This module, originally oriented toward ambulatory care, was expanded to form the basis for a system-wide clinical data repository.

Technical infrastructure also required considerable expansion.

EHR systems functionality was built through a PCE application that captured data needed for a longitudinal patient record. PCE contained data from ancillary packages, such as laboratory, pharmacy, and radiology, as well as clinician interactive applications, such as the problem list, progress notes, and medical imaging.

The PCE module provided health maintenance alerts and reminders covering 16 common outpatient conditions. An electronic mail package and sharing of problem list, progress notes, and discharge summary information supported communications related to patient care.

Data entry could be provided by clerical and clinical staff. Routine access to DHCP applications was available to clinicians and other users 24 hours a day, 7 days a week as a function of their level of security and menu options they had been provided. Because more than 10 percent of VHA patients received care at more than one facility, interfacility data access was achieved through the patient data exchange. DHCP usage was pervasive organization-wide.

TECHNOLOGY

Due to VHA's overall strategy to implement cost-effective systems that make the best use of all available resources and technologies, the basic DHCP hospital system was built on existing industry standards and layered software. This allowed the VA to achieve maximum portability and vendor independence.

For example, DHCP was developed in an American National Standards Institute (ANSI) standard language and database management system [Massachusetts General Hospital Utility Multi-Programming System (M or MUMPS)], the Kernel operating system. This enabled DHCP applications to run unmodified on hardware as diverse as a fax and a PC under operating systems as different as virtual memory system (VMS), UNIX, and DOS. Platform independent, DHCP thus was extremely flexible and scalable in its hardware requirements.

Hardware architecture in 1994 was focused on a central processing cluster comprised of a tightly coupled network of 486 systems in the 60 smallest sites or four to six Digital Equipment Corporation (DEC) Alpha systems in the large 100-plus sites. The data modeling approach used was governed by VA FileMan, which implemented a hybrid hierarchical network model with some relational properties.

DHCP's track record for extensibility in response to technological change was superlative, enabling extension to client/server application modules, incorporation of microcomputer workstations, and the introduction of transmission control protocol/Internet protocol (TCP/IP) as a protocol for electronic mail transfer.

VALUE

In 1994, formal studies of EHR impact on quality of care were not commonplace in VHA due to the absence of a formal structure and staff to support such studies. Efforts were being made, however, to increase evaluation of clinical packages. For example, one project was being launched to assess the effectiveness of preventive care alerts, and another to assess the impact of PCE on the primary clinic's ability to enhance patient access to care.

VHA used the quality improvement checklist (QUIC) application, designed to enhance its accountability within a framework of continuous quality improvement, using system-wide comparative data to analyze and enhance healthcare services. VHA was identifying and putting in place evaluation measures for quality, including those contributing to the assessment of whether care was needed, was competent or not, and was cost effective.

Internal studies to assess the cost impact of the DHCP had not yet been conducted. However, a 1992 study by the Office of the Inspector General for the Department of Veterans Affairs provided indirect evidence of the impact of DHCP. That study concluded: "A comparison of total effort and expenditures of 16 carefully matched pairs of major VAMCs and their affiliated state university teaching hospitals shows that VAMC costs per equivalent work unit were approximately 60 percent that of comparable university hospitals."

1995 DAVIES ORGANIZATIONAL AWARD WINNER
INTERMOUNTAIN HEALTHCARE

ABOUT THE ORGANIZATION

More than 40 years ago, a visionary group of clinicians and scientists at LDS (Latter-day Saints) Hospital in Salt Lake City, Utah, began applying computer technology to patient care. From these early experiments arose an integrated, patient-centered, rules-based CIS called Health Evaluation through Logical Processing (HELP). While its creation was remarkable, the acceptance it received from caregivers was truly impressive.

Concurrent with the development of HELP, Intermountain Healthcare (IHC), LDS Hospital's parent corporation, was forming. This 15-hospital, not-for-profit system, which was donated by the Church of Jesus Christ of Latter-day Saints, served communities in Utah and Southeastern Idaho. An EHR was critical to its success as an integrated, regional healthcare delivery system.

After working through the 1950s and 1960s at LDS Hospital to automate clinical departments, HELP was created from the vision of Dr. Homer R. Warner and his colleagues. They wanted an integrated, comprehensive, patient-focused database to give caregivers a comprehensive view of patient data; and to apply rules-based logic to patient data permitting unsolicited patient-specific reminders and alerts to caregivers to facilitate uniform, consistent, quality care.

With the financial support of hospital leadership and with academic support from the University of Utah, the LDS Hospital Department of Medical Biophysics and Computing began the collaboration among clinicians and computer scientists to create the HELP system.

MANAGEMENT

Throughout the late 1970s and early 1980s, while HELP was expanding its clinical presence at LDS Hospital, IHC continued to develop as a multi-hospital delivery system. By 1985, IHC recognized the pressing need for a system-wide EHR. To make this a reality, IHC adopted the following planning and organizational processes:

- Creation of an Information Systems Committee of the Corporate Board of Trustees to provide ongoing strategic focus;
- Provision of a five-year budget of $50 million;
- Establishment of organizational linkages for coordination and integrated leadership between IHC's Information Systems department and medical informatics;
- Creation of a newsletter to inform and involve clinicians;
- Project renaming as IHCNet to maintain focus on the IHC-wide network fostering integration; and
- Full organizational support for IHC's common enterprise-wide voice/data network.

Following board approval to broadly install HELP, information systems leadership chose strategies to minimize risk. IHC reached a joint development agreement with 3M Health Information Systems to broaden HELP technologically and functionally. The system purchased and installed a commercial laboratory computer system, rather than building the system, to reduce internal development resources. A dedicated IHC-wide voice/data network was formed with vendor agreements for switch, T1 line and microwave services.

IHC selected McKay-Dee Medical Center, a 360-bed regional facility in Ogden, Utah, as HELP's first pilot beyond LDS Hospital. A computer training room with PCs and demonstration software was set up for 20 staff at a time, and IHC placed a medical informatics specialist at McKay-Dee for physician training.

The Informatics Council of IHC coordinated general review of system performance, policies and user feedback. Consisting of medical informatics specialists from the central office and each hospital, the council met regularly to coordinate installations, support, and training.

Key to the success of the project was a guarantee data residing in the EHR was high quality. Only data critical to patient care was collected. Data was recorded at the point of care in real time. The EHR was the clinical record for each patient; all data was linked to the responsible caregiver. To reduce entry errors, the HELP system supported several quality validation functions, including data entry field level validity/range/domain checks, consistency checks between fields, and HELP validation logic.

To measure project benefits, IHC conducted physician and nurse surveys, and special studies. Physician testimonials, ongoing modifications to reflect improvement initiatives and the lack of turnover in project leadership were critical success factors.

FUNCTIONALITY

IHC planned its EHR according to the needs of five major categories of users: healthcare providers, patients, administrators, third-party payors, and researchers. These users would rely upon the EHR for direct patient care, administration and management, reimbursement, and research. The EHR's role as data repository was central to each user group.

HELP maintained a site-specific, encounter-based EHR for each hospital. A WAN linking all IHC facilities enabled real-time consolidation of data from individual sites. Key to HELP was its integrated computerized medical record that contained information from the laboratory, pharmacy, nursing, surgery, intensive care, medical records, and other locations.

To support the complex data collection requirements of HELP, authorized users could create new data variables, design data collection screens, and store this information.

Entry screens and logical rules that flagged or blocked inappropriate entries for certain fields helped to ensure quality data and enhance data accuracy. Data screens on the HELP system employed error checking and range checking to verify accuracy. Selection lists, with limited choices, reduced errors.

IHC assembled multi-disciplinary and multi-facility teams of physicians, nurses, and other providers to determine the core data elements to be collected. This process ensured data was useful across disciplines and facilities.

IHC designed several features to increase efficiency. First, the EHR avoided data redundancy through one-time data entry. A single data dictionary was established; it was maintained in a central setting and controlled all data collected by HELP. The EHR maintained financial and cost information to facilitate administrative functions, eliminating traditional paper documents like lab and shift reports.

One of HELP's key features was its ability to provide online clinical decision assistance. An expert-maintained knowledge base contained rules and statistics to monitor data and decisions made on a patient. Activation of the knowledge base was either automatic as data was stored in the EHR or on demand by the user to evaluate a decision questioned by the application.

TECHNOLOGY

The HELP system ran primarily on hardware from Tandem. At the time of the Davies Award, LDS Hospital used a 12-CPU system with 64 megabytes (MB) of random access memory (RAM) per processor and 14 gigabytes (GB) of disk space. Simple VT100 serial terminals were replaced with PC-type workstations to achieve a client/server environment. At LDS, HELP communicated with users through approximately 1,200 workstations and 200 strategically located laser printers.

Fiber optic cabling connected between floors and across long distances. The majority of workstations communicated over the hospital's LAN. IHC's WAN linked facilities using microwave, T1 and T3 capabilities.

HELP software was a combination of tools and applications developed as part of the partnership between IHC and 3M. Encoded data was the core of most reports, decision-making, and other functions of HELP. Information was maintained in a tightly coded form for flexible review by clinicians and for storage. Free text reports were a significant part of medical records, x-ray reports, documented histories, physical examinations, operative reports, and discharge summaries. Analog data was managed through interfaces with outside systems. Interpretations were communicated to HELP where they were encoded for decision support.

The encoding system was called point-to-text (PTXT). PTXT consisted of a medical dictionary and a mechanism for storing groups of terms in a compressed form in the patient database. Medical concepts, represented by text, were linked to eight-byte codes.

User applications were created using an interpreted, high-level language, PTXT application language (PAL), designed specifically for medical use. As HELP evolved, its developers incorporated into PAL and its underlying system routines, special functionality to aid medical decisions.

From its inception, security and the integrity of clinical data were a high priority for HELP. Only those with authorized passwords were allowed access. An audit trail of what each user entered was kept to deter and police unauthorized access. For security, the HELP system data entry and review structure focused on data from a single patient. An aggressive Security and Confidentiality Committee was in place.

The Tandem hardware was setup so each CPU and its controllers had a backup processor. Every disk drive featured a primary copy and a mirrored copy. As a result, the system was operational 24 hours per day, seven days per week.

IHC continually measured up time and response time statistics. System availability was consistently 99.8 percent, a downtime of less than three minutes per day. Using response time information, IHC worked to improve software, hardware capability, and communications strategies. Efficiency was emphasized in the more frequently used reports, for example, and IHC upgraded to faster reduced instruction set computer (RISC) processors and fiber optic Ethernet LANs.

VALUE

The availability of accurate, timely patient information contributed significantly to improvements in patient care. HELP addressed pharmacy alerts, alerts based on abnormal laboratory results, respiratory care, the use of blood products, infectious disease monitoring and antibiotic use, monitoring of adverse drug events, and the treatment of adult respiratory distress syndrome.

During 1989, LDS Hospital had more than 20,000 inpatients who received approximately 1.3 million medication doses. There were 703 action-oriented medication alerts; physicians responded to all.

Laboratory results in HELP were used to develop an alert system for life-threatening conditions leading to an increase in the proportion of patients who received appropriate care—50.8 percent before implementation versus 62.5 percent afterwards.

The HELP system generated cost savings. To begin with, in an 18-month period, only nine adverse drug events were reported using manual mechanisms. During the same time interval, 731 adverse events were detected and verified by computer methods—an 80-fold increase. IHC found prevention and early treatment reduced the length of hospitalization, bringing cost savings and reducing mortality.

IHC found HELP to be a useful tool for screening adult acute care patients for inappropriate days of care. Estimates indicated in a capitated healthcare marketplace IHC would save $500,000 to $1,000,000 annually by identifying patients inappropriately hospitalized.

A key feature of HELP was its evaluation of medication orders for drug interactions. Pharmacists notified physicians when the computer indicated an inappropriate medication. Physician compliance went from approximately 70 percent to virtually 100 percent. Over a two-year period of study, 2,100 drug alerts were generated, achieving a benefit to cost ratio of 3.98. The HELP system was used extensively for research and epidemiology in quality of care issues as well as research into the science of medical computing.

With a pioneering spirit, IHC leaders stepped boldly into the development and growth of a working EHR. They affirmed HELP had, "over the years, become a critical infrastructure at LDS Hospital in support of world-class patient care."

1996 DAVIES ORGANIZATIONAL AWARD WINNER
BRIGHAM AND WOMEN'S HOSPITAL

ABOUT THE ORGANIZATION

Brigham and Women's Hospital (BWH) is a more than 700-bed academic medical center in Boston, Massachusetts. At the time it won the Davies Award in 1996, BWH admitted 36,000 inpatients and provided care to 600,000-plus outpatients each year at four sites.

In 1989, BWH began a major initiative to redevelop its information system. The goals were to establish a new technical platform that would support the hospital's continuing expansion, and to build new CIS focused on medical logic interventions that prevent adverse events, reduce the cost of care, and guide caregivers to optimal care processes.

Called the Brigham Integrated Computing System (BICS), it organized clinical data, including specimen laboratory and patients studies, into logical information displays, combining information from disparate sources for the caregiver's benefit. BICS originally included registration, admit/discharge, and financial information; laboratory, specimen, and pathology results; test x-ray, EKG, and procedure reports; and dictated discharge summaries and operative notes. Other functions added in subsequent years included a full ambulatory medical record and inpatient interim summaries (sign-out information). In 1996, BICS had 4,500 clients connected to the network; 8,000 users accessed the system, averaging 25,000 log-ins daily.

MANAGEMENT

The BICS development and implementation benefited from four significant management factors.

First, the project had strong support from senior management and medical staff, who, as a result of practical experience and ongoing education, believed in the power of information technology to improve the quality of care while reducing its costs.

Second, organizational precursors supported BICS development. Precursors included coherent and intelligent organizational strategies related to mission, service and market position, performance measurement, and process improvement; effective internal communication; strong medical staff leadership; and good working relationships between administration, nursing, and the medical staff. Other precursors included interdisciplinary team-based experience with process improvement, a solid core set of data, and a solid applications and technology platform.

Third, a well-conceived care quality improvement structure was already in place at BWH. Organization of the effort to support BICS included a Care Improvement Council, a Clinical Initiatives Development Program, the Center for Applied Medical Information Systems Research, knowledge domain committees, and information systems development and support staff.

Fourth, the hospital consistently used an internal application development strategy, which closely paired developers with users, employed rapid prototyping, and implemented an application as soon as it had sufficient useful functionality. Implementation benefited from thorough consideration of user needs and practicing clinician input during the design, introduction, and roll-out phases. Once applications were established, users received continuing support.

FUNCTIONALITY

BICS' functional objectives were as follows:
- To store and make available to all caregivers as much relevant clinical information as possible, with an emphasis on data that could be encoded and used for care and decision support;
- To ensure programs and screens emphasized logical information display;
- To feature appropriate interventions that provided caregivers with information to modify the current process of care;
- To permit efficient communication of data from one caregiver to another; and
- To provide advanced services and displays that enhanced the convenience, education, and general satisfaction of the user.

The BICS ambulatory record, which replaced the paper chart, was designed to support the most frequent clinical scenarios. It contained problem lists, progress notes, medications and allergies, vital signs, pending to-do items, and health maintenance information. Because the operation of the record followed the same standards as the rest of the system, no special training was required for the ambulatory application. Formal BICS system training required for physicians and nurses was minimal, involving only a 45-minute group introduction to order entry and basic system operation. After, clinicians used the system independently.

Following the initiation of computerized practitioner order entry (CPOE), built in house and released in 1993, all orders on all adult inpatients services were entered through BICS. Universal access to workstations reduced the number of verbal orders. Assisted-mode, template-based screens, designed for each type of order, whether for medications, laboratory tests, or others, prompted users for required fields.

Order sets and templates were used when a clinical situation called for a group of orders that were often ordered together. Physicians could create and use their own personal order sets at any time, but these sets remained private. (The use of private order sets were discontinued in 2001 due to concerns they could lead to unsafe practices; approved order sets remain and account for a substantial percentage of all orders.) Default doses and frequencies established by the hospital pharmacy reminded clinicians of standard practice right at the time of ordering. The system provided alerts, warnings, and other ordering suggestions. By displaying the charges assessed for laboratory tests and radiology procedures, BICS helped to promote hospital policies and cost-conscious care.

An event engine was designed to sense unusual events triggered by an occurrence, such as the entry of new data (for example, a critically abnormal lab result) or the passage of time, to test such events for importance to the patient and to rapidly convey enough information to the caregiver so swift action could be taken in response. The

BICS Sign-Out and Coverage List systems allowed caregivers to efficiently communicate relevant patient information to the caregiver who was providing off-hours coverage. An automated department log and an expect log enabled the emergency department to track and improve patient flow.

TECHNOLOGY

The technological development of BICS is a story of development of one of the largest client server systems in healthcare. Achieved with minimal disturbance of function, this involved the conversion of an existing minicomputer-based system to a new network platform based on MUMPS and personal computers. Conversion to the new platform occurred in three phases: analysis and prototype, limited deployment, and full deployment.

In 1996, BICS ran on a network of more than 6,000 personal computers and handled more than 40,000 sign-ons daily. New BICS applications used a windowed user interface (Hyper-M), which was keyboard or mouse controlled. The system was available 24 hours a day. On inpatients units, there were five workstations per 15-bed units; in intensive care areas, one station served one or two beds. Workstations were located on all inpatient floors, in all ambulatory practices, most business offices, and other strategic locations. Dedicated copper and fiber optic cable connected off-site facilities and clinical sites of the hospital's primary health maintenance organization (HMO).

The network's physical structure was two-tiered: local departmental rings communicated with other rings through a second tier with two backbone rings, one for MUMPS-based applications, and the other for DOS-based PC applications. System software applications were developed in, or converted to, DataTree MUMPS (DTM, now InterSystems Cache).

Network management controls were available at the application, network operating system, and wire levels. Each MUMPS server had a shadow backup that constantly maintained an exact copy of the server's databases on its own disk. Access to BICS was controlled by a password and by authorizations to the various application menus.

Design lessons included how to take full advantage of the scalability benefits of client/server architecture. This could be achieved by ensuring as much processing as possible occurred on the client. BWH learned organizations should be able to split databases and server-based application processing across multiple servers and transferability across other settings, both small and large, could be achieved.

VALUE

The measurement and analysis of BICS impact benefited from BWH's active program in health services research and epidemiology, which focused on the study of care processes, adverse events and their preventability, and patient outcomes. Before-and-after studies and randomized controlled trials of interventions that affected ordering patterns and other elements of care delivery were extensive. Patient safety, care outcomes, and cost impact were thoroughly documented.

For example, the 1,500 annual allergy warnings provided to clinicians through BICS had an identified potential to prevent 40 adverse events per year. Seventy percent of orders carrying allergy warnings were canceled by the clinician who ordered after receipt of the warning, resulting in an estimated cost savings of $250,000.

Response to clinical interventions was often dramatic post BICS implementation. For example, use of favored H2 blockers changed from 4 percent to 94 percent within a week of that intervention's introduction. Inpatient admissions with un-cosigned orders after discharge fell from 80 percent to 5 percent.

As a side effect of the process changes introduced with BICS, lax processes were identified and improved. For example, when order entry was introduced, a large number of orders were staying unacknowledged on one unit's monitor, suggesting the nurse was taking a long time to review new orders. Examination of the process indicated orders on the floor were viewed first by the unit secretary, who would contact the nurse if any orders needed nursing attention. New processes were instituted to codify when this mode of operation was appropriate or not.

The presence of advanced information systems provided a strategic advantage as well. BICS was offered as an incentive for off-site physician groups interested in referring their patients to BWH. The scientific and educational impact of BICS was significant. Patients received tailored discharge instructions, and both patients and providers could obtain a wide range of educational materials.

Management of the introduction of CIS at BWH benefited from bottom-line characteristics that made BICS successful. BWH management and clinicians viewed CIS as part of a collection of tools for improving the quality and reducing the cost of care, and they thoughtfully approached information system implementation as an organizational process.

"Without these characteristics—clinically-focused design and emphasis on care improvement, early adoption of modern technologies, strong support of users, and a supportive, well-organized management structure—it would have been far more difficult to realize the favorable impact BICS has had at our hospital," concludes the BICS management team.

EVOLUTION OF THE ORGANIZATION, ITS EHR, AND LESSONS TO SHARE

Challenges Created by Organizational Evolution

Concurrent with and following development of the initial Davies Award application, BWH experienced major organizational change, becoming part of Partners Healthcare System. Initially formed in 1994 through the merger of BWH and Massachusetts General Hospital (MGH), Partners Healthcare System expanded since that time to include 10 hospitals and an extended network of ambulatory providers. The information systems departments of BWH and MGH were consolidated in 1996.

Partners Healthcare System hospitals are greatly varied in size, location (urban or rural), affiliations (academic and non-academic), patient populations, and most significantly, governance models. The same is true for the affiliated ambulatory practices.

This posed significant challenges for the organization and for information systems. The differing cultures of each institution required different approaches to readiness assessment, technology planning, and implementation strategy. However, it was and continues to be in Partners' best interest to minimize the rework required to implement comparable functionalities at different sites.

Information systems, thus, undertook a multi-year strategy process to improve its capabilities in this new multi-site vendor role, taking on industry-based functions such as product management.

The evolution of Partners also placed new demands on technology and functionality standardization, which led to a number of projects, including the following:

- **Common data repository:** This single place to store and display information from many different sources requires reconciliation and normalization of data vocabularies from different systems.
- **Master patient index:** This single, unique index includes patients from all Partners sites.
- **Allergy normalization:** A common list and vocabulary serve all CIS that store or work with patient drug allergies and sensitivities.
- **Knowledge management:** A comprehensive list of rules, information resources and other clinical decision support content, and plans to offer common, non-conflicting decision support at all Partners sites.

Changing Technology and Functionality

At the time of the 1996 Davies monograph, plans were already underway to make extensive use of evolving Windows and Web technologies. Partners-wide applications, such as the common results viewer, and MGH versions of applications such as CPOE and the ambulatory record (now called the longitudinal medical record or LMR), were developed in Windows in the mid-1990s.

The new version of the online reference library, handbook, became the first Web-based system. The LMR and results viewer made the jump to Web technologies in the late 1990s and early 2000s. Most new applications are now developed using Web browser technologies, and are also available off site through the Partners virtual private network (VPN).

At this time, most but not all Partners hospitals feed data into the common repository, and the LMR is the standard ambulatory record for BWH, MGH, and several hundred ambulatory clinicians. Other hospitals and practices use a variety of commercial systems.

CPOE was redeveloped using Windows technologies (primarily Visual Basic and Visual C++) for the MGH inpatient service, while BWH continues to use the Hyper-M version. A distinct version of CPOE was developed for the BWH emergency department, similar to the MGH inpatient system but with key differences such as automatic order set selection based on the chief complaint. CPOE extensions were also developed for chemotherapy protocols.

The BWH neonatal service, the only service not using CPOE after 1995, went live with CPOE in 2004, after extensive work to accommodate the special drug dosing and therapies unique to neonatal care. In 2005, BWH went live with an electronic medication administration record (eMAR), which has already shown promise in reducing medication delivery errors just as CPOE has reduced ordering errors.

Other functions and important features added since 1996 include:

- Picture archiving and communication system (PACS) and EKG systems to store and present graphic and image data;
- Automatic discharge summaries generated from inpatient data and sign-out information;
- Expansion of the event engine to handle multi-step algorithms, adverse event detection, automatic prompts for communication with referring physicians, and more;
- Emergency medicine systems, including advanced patient tracking, alerts about a variety of time-sensitive events, and clinical documentation;
- Further expansion of the handbook, including more commercial reference sources and the use of KnowledgeLinks, first developed at Partners in 1998. The KnowledgeLinks' capabilities allow a user to enter a single search string and content type, and obtain pertinent material from the most relevant available reference source. KnowledgeLinks are usually used as info buttons right in the EHR, letting users get relevant information as they enter or review data; and
- Patient Gateway, which commencing in 1997 provided access to health knowledge for patients on Partners' public Web site. Information was organized by condition type and by type of knowledge or action, allowing patients to find the information that best answered their current questions. Since 2001, patient interface functions greatly expanded and development has moved toward facilitating the patient-physician relationship. Patients can now use Patient Gateway to communicate with their clinicians, schedule appointments, validate referrals, and more.

The EHR's Continued Effect on Healthcare

BWH and Partners have been at the very forefront of health services research nationally and internationally. Extensive research has been conducted on the impact of CIS developed at BWH and Partners as a whole. The organization's systems have provided some of the largest care-improvement benefits evidenced to date.

As a result, information technology has occupied an ever-increasing role as a major tool in quality improvement programs. Partners established five signature initiatives in 2003, reflecting five core areas of focus system-wide: maximizing the use of new clinical information technology; increasing patient safety and reducing medical errors; making high quality patient care uniform across the Partners system; coordinating care for patients with high cost diseases; and improving efficiency in the use of prescription drugs and radiology procedures. All of these initiatives involve major information systems contributions, and the first core area is exclusively about clinical systems expansion. Further projects have concentrated on the safety and quality impact of several new technologies implemented at BWH, including e-prescribing, eMAR, chemotherapy information systems, and event detection.

Information Systems-related health services research at BWH also focuses on understanding the nature and incidence of errors, adverse events, excess costs, and inefficiencies in a variety of settings of care, and the potential for information systems to improve the current state. A new organization arising from Partners information systems, the Center for Information Technology Leadership, produced several widely read analyses of the value equation for health information technologies, including ambulatory CPOE and health information exchange, and interoperability.

The department of radiology has developed a CPOE add-on that provides critical advice on optimal radiology test usage during the ordering process.

Through a newly funded genomics center based at Children's Hospital Boston and extensive use of information technologies, Partners promises to add another new dimension to patient care by analyzing the clinical impact of genetic variations among individuals.

Recognizing the convergence between information gathering and optimal use of the vast medical knowledge base, in 2005, Harvard Medical School named two well-known medical informatics experts to direct Harvard's Countway Library of Medicine.

These initiatives are examples of the value-related lessons of the BICS project, which spurred further system development and use throughout Partners Healthcare System.

Lessons to Share

Although BWH and Partners, like some other early Davies Award winners, have achieved great success with a homegrown system, the organization's leaders indicate this is probably not the recommended path for a new organization. "Homegrown systems allow greater customization to local needs, of course, but the time and effort required to build up an organization, develop the system, and provide effective customer service are enormous," they note. "BICS and its descendants were developed internally because effective commercial solutions were simply not available at the time. Once the foundation was built, further development was less of an additive task. Current-day commercial CIS for inpatient and ambulatory use are plentiful and provide substantial functionality." Their additional lessons to be shared follow.

Two functional cornerstones of EHRs have high impact on safety, quality, and efficiency: easy, comprehensive access to data, and extensive, effective clinical decision support. Adoption of the latter is still an inexact science. Several U.S. healthcare organizations have implemented electronic records but turned off clinical decision support functions for fear of introducing too much complexity.

The system must be recognized as a friend to the clinician right from the start, but it is equally important to keep clinical decision support high in the priority list. Choose a set of non-threatening, highly-valued clinical decision support functions for initial implementation (for example, allergy warnings, dose recommendations), and then add more complex decision support as the system becomes more established.

Both strategic goals for an EHR system implementation and marketing the system by noting its progress toward those goals are critical. Choose goals that are clinical (not technological), easy to understand by the whole organization, and that if achieved will be a source of pride to the organization. Communicate the goals widely, put extra effort into achieving them, and publish frequent progress reports in the organization's communications vehicles.

Finally, understand the people processes and real relationships in the organization, and overdo inclusion and early, honest communication. These steps are easily as important as good system design in ensuring a successful implementation.

1996 DAVIES ORGANIZATIONAL AWARD WINNER
GROUP HEALTH COOPERATIVE OF PUGET SOUND

The first portion of this chapter describes an EHR system that Group Health Cooperative (GHC) developed and implemented on a pilot basis in the early 1990s. The organization won a Davies Organizational Award of Excellence in 1996 for this initiative, named the Clinically Related Information System (CRIS) project.

The second portion of this chapter, Group Health Cooperative's EHR Today, describes GHC's recent implementation of an EHR/Patient Access system both organization-wide and significantly, membership-wide. Note GHC's leaders, "This system is one of the most far- reaching EHR projects in the world with more than 105,000 patients online, accessing their medical records, and communicating with their physicians online across Washington and North Idaho."

ABOUT THE ORGANIZATION

In 1996, Group Health Cooperative of Puget Sound (GHC) was a consumer-governed, health maintenance organization in Washington. At the time it won the Davies Award, GHC was the sixth largest non-profit HMO in the nation with more than 500,000 members to whom it provided care through 30 primary care sites, two hospitals, five specialty centers, a nurse facility, and a community home health division.

In 1996, GHC used a staff model in which physicians were employed by the HMO. Members choose a primary care physician from among those on the staff. Each full-time family practice physician, assisted by nurse practitioners, physician's assistants, registered nurses, and other allied professionals, was responsible for a panel of 1,500 to 2,000 patients. Specialty care was provided by both staff and contracted specialists upon referral from the family practice physician.

GHC looked (and continues to look) at its patients—also known as consumers or members—not just as individuals, but as members of groups with shared health needs. This population-based approach to managing and delivering healthcare is designed, organized, and funded on the basis of specific patient groupings that share a defined geography, clinical need, or demographic characteristic, such as age or sex.

MANAGEMENT

Planning for an automated patient record that would be available in a timely manner at the point of care began in the late 1980s. Called the CRIS project, its goals were to improve the health of patients, patient and provider satisfaction, and to lower costs of care.

Identified through focus groups and medical staff surveys, two critical user requirements provided the backbone for CRIS goals:
• Clinician tools aimed at improving individual patient care and helping clinicians understand, manage, and improve the healthcare of the entire patient population.

Thus, a patient problem list and the ability to identify and list individuals with a particular problem were key requirements.

• Advice rules for clinicians that would fire automatically when reviewing an individual patient and could be run for an entire panel of patients.

Recognizing there were no acceptable commercial products available to meet these two requirements, GHC built its own EHR system. It piloted the system in one medical center for one primary care team with five full-time or part-time team members. The goal of the prototype initiative was to transfer learning about clinical process redesign, and database and screen design to an organization-wide system. GHC expected technology to change by the time it was ready for organization-wide implementation.

A physician/nurse user team wrote and prioritized advice rules in six clinical areas: breast and colorectal cancer screening, smoking cessation, sedentary-life lifestyle, type 2 diabetes mellitus care, childhood and adult immunizations, and monitoring patients treated with warfarin and digoxin. Nineteen small computer programs were written to cover the advice rules requirement.

Development, testing, and installation of the prototype system and staff training occurred from the summer of 1992 through the summer of 1993. GHC conducted both user acceptance testing and system testing covering performance, volume, functionality, and security. Technology and functionality refinements occurred in 1993 and 1994.

In late 1995, after two and a half years of use, the prototype was dismantled due to its increasing maintenance costs and the transfer of resources to development of an organization-wide solution.

FUNCTIONALITY

In addition to improved access to necessary information for clinical decision-making, criteria for EHR functionality included providing tools for communicating with consumers, providing a balance between enough and too much data, and improving communication and planning among the healthcare team members. Provider surveys identified the problem list and the advice rules as the major value-added aspects of an EHR.

Specific CRIS functionality included demographic information, problem list, current medication list, prioritized advice rules (with the highest priority advice rule popping up automatically), and the ability to look up laboratory and anatomic pathology results, visit histories, immunization history, and breast cancer screening data. The results-reporting functionality enhanced the functionality then available organization-wide by allowing the entry of the member's number only once for any of the look-up and results-reporting transactions.

Advice rules supported by CRIS included, among others, breast and colon cancer screening, diabetes management, hypertension management, drug therapy complications, and immunizations.

TECHNOLOGY

Using a structured project management process, the CRIS EHR team identified how the individual workstation and EHR data availability would fit into the center's work flow and how data flow documents could clarify the design and management of EHR development tasks.

The basic architecture of the system called for a nightly extraction of data from existing organization-wide laboratory, pharmacy, visits, and consumer databases and placement in a new relational structured query language (SQL) server-based database. Eight workstations in the medical center offices and exam rooms were connected to GHC's mainframe. The advice rule programming used SQL server's stored procedure capability. The GUI used Microsoft Visual Basic System maintenance took only a small part of one database administrator's time.

VALUE

Instituting an EHR proved to be a far more complex task than simply changing the medium upon which the patient's data resided. User team members spent additional time to review and act on the new information available to them and had to define new roles. However, they found new ways of working together, and began to make care decisions for entire groups of patients, rather than ad hoc one-by-one decisions for individual patients.

Quality of care indicators, centered on the rate of compliance with cancer screening, immunization completeness, and implementation of warfarin monitoring rules, increased in a positive direction following implementation of the EHR. In addition, the EHR enforced the use of the problem list by including an automatic link between each problem and the encounter date.

Although development and installation costs were higher than expected, the cost impact was at least in part offset by the benefits of improved preventive care services. The ability to review an entire panel of warfarin results at the same time, or to mail mammography reminders simultaneously to all patients, was clearly superior to doing it one by one.

Health status of the population served and patient satisfaction remained essentially the same pre- and post-EHR implementation. However, provider satisfaction improved significantly, from a 50 percent satisfaction rate with the overall quality of care providers were able to provide (satisfied or very satisfied) to 100 percent satisfaction. The regular team meetings required to implement the CRIS system helped to clarify and establish a common philosophy of care. Over time, team meetings became data driven, discussion centered on how to modify routines to improve care, and the process of monitoring compliance provided a very positive experience for all team members.

In addition, CRIS EHR implementation contributed to research on issues of implementation of guidelines, expansion of preventive care practices, increased efficiency at the primary care site, and use of mid-level providers.

In summarizing the benefits of the CRIS pilot project, GHC's leaders indicated the project served "yeoman's duty" as a functioning prototype for an organization-wide EHR: "It reinforced our goal of designing an EHR not for how healthcare is practiced today, but for the way we want healthcare to be practiced in the future. This meant keeping a firm grasp on the need for population management in addition to individual patient management."

GROUP HEALTH COOPERATIVE AND ITS EHR TODAY

The Organization

GHC is a much different organization in 2006, than it was in 1996, and its name, simply Group Health Cooperative (Group Health) reflects the transformation. Group Health is now a group model non-profit health system covering the entire state of Washington and North Idaho. As the nation's second-largest consumer-governed healthcare organization, Group Health now has 580,000 members (this includes subsidiary health carriers, GHC Options Inc. and KPS Health Plans), 70 percent of whom receive care in Group Health-owned facilities. Its mission is to design, deliver, and finance high-quality healthcare.

In addition to the types of facilities mentioned earlier, Group Health now includes behavioral health clinics, vision centers, auditory rehabilitation centers, and speech, language and learning services centers. The organization has a staff of approximately 9,600, including more than 800 physicians, and achieves more than 1.4 million patient encounters on an annual basis.

Objectives of New EHR System

Group Health initiated its CIS EHR project in the early 2000s in order to create significant clinical and business process transformation to improve the delivery of high-quality, customer- focused, cost-effective care at Group Health and in the healthcare industry; and to emphasize Group Health's market differentiation as an innovative and patient-focused healthcare organization.

The CIS was intended to include:
- An automated tool for the provision and documentation of care to Group Health patients at the point of care regardless of where, when, or how the care is delivered;
- A longitudinal patient record and clinical repository; and
- A comprehensive patient online medical record to include secure e-mail access to every care provider, access to lab and test results, allergy information, immunizations on demand, visit summaries, and a trajectory to full medical record transparency.

The vision for Group Health's secure patient Internet portal, MyGroupHealth (www.ghc.org), was to "create an experience that enables unparalleled access and transparency for Group Health's customers by connecting members, staff, community providers, purchasers, and brokers with Group Health and with one another at the right place and the right time." Group Health would build its electronic medical record (EMR) as one that is owned by patients and physicians together, and would use this approach to guide every design decision made in new development and maintenance of the installation.

Group Health achieved these objectives and vision.

EHR System and Implementation

Group Health chose Epic Systems Corporation's EpicCare product suite. Specific EpicCare components installed included EpicCare Ambulatory (physician order entry, documentation, messaging, and clinical data repository), MyChart (secure patient access to physicians for e-mail, lab and test results, immunizations, allergy information, and after visit summaries), Clarity (enterprise reporting), and MyEpic (secure report distribution).

Group Health patients were prioritized as the key users and coauthors of the EHR from the beginning. Group Health was the first and only Epic Systems client to roll out its EHR product to patients (July 2003) before it was rolled out to providers (approximately one year later). On August 14, 2003, the patient online medical record was made available across Washington via MyGroupHealth. This was called the "big bang." Every patient generated e-mail is filed in the electronic chart along with physician progress notes, and the default for most aspects of the clinical record is full sharing.

Following this event, roll out of provider components, including order entry, documentation, decision support, and reporting began. From the start, providers used the EHR with the idea the record would be shared, and the customer service value of an automated health record was established organization-wide. Implementation at practice sites was completed by the end of 2005.

Group Health is a pioneer in Information Therapy, which joins clinical data on the Web with relevant patient information from the Healthwise® Knowledgebase. The result is the online medical record becomes the ultimate search engine for Group Health members accessing their medical record information online.

Clinical Decision Support

Group Health has an active clinical decision support infrastructure, with several tiers of guidance available. Ordering and documentation templates are based on evidence-based principles. More active decision support is also in place, in the form of alternative drug alerts, interaction and allergy alerts, and best-practice alerts. Alternative drug alerts are designed to inform physicians of therapeutically equivalent medications with improved cost profiles. These alerts allow clinicians to use professional judgment in accepting alternatives. The best-practice alerts use the most current knowledge about factors for success in clinical decision support systems.

As with the design of the entire system, alerts are intended to guide physicians and patients to the most effective, affordable care. Alerts incorporate links to supportive documentation, including patient education, and are designed to be read by patients as well as providers in exam rooms.

Value

Group Health's leaders indicate that CIS/MyGroupHealth project is one of the most successful Group Health has ever undertaken, in terms of its transformation of the organization, and impact on members and providers. Its value as a tool is not strictly cost reduction; it is improvement in the quality of service, quality of care, and efficiency of the care system.

Lessons Learned

The Group Health CIS team can point to several critical success factors in achieving its goals. The first and most important is the treatment of this project as a business and clinical transformation project rather than an information technology project. Functional teams were involved in understanding the process of care and patient experience from the start of the work, and continue to focus on outcomes in that area to this day. Team members are skilled in diagramming work flows and working with care system leaders to optimize these over time.

Physician leadership and partnership was also critical; direction provided by the Medical Group through a medical director of informatics was and is used continuously to guide the design of new features and upgrades to the system.

It is also clear from Group Health's experience there is tremendous value in putting the patient at the center of all activities related to EHR implementation. Group Health's member-governed status ensures the patient is always thought of as the primary customer of everything the organization does.

Group Health's leaders conclude, "Our team was pleased to be able to carry this idea into implementation with us. At Group Health, the CIS is a tool used to deliver high-quality, affordable care, which includes excellent customer service and care at the convenience of the patient. Our adoption of a comprehensive patient and physician accessible EMR is one of the most transformational activities in our history."

1997 DAVIES ORGANIZATIONAL AWARD WINNER
KAISER PERMANENTE OF OHIO

ABOUT THE ORGANIZATION

In 1989, the Kaiser Health Plan of Ohio—with leadership from the Ohio Permanente Medical Group, its principal provider of medical care—formed a team of management, information systems and medical staff representatives to explore the status of clinical information systems (CIS) around the country. Allan Khoury, MD, lead physician, proposed building an Encounter System, a semi-automated medical record, to complement the paper chart.

By 1994, Kaiser Permanente of Ohio began planning for the Medical Automated Record System (MARS), the successor to the Encounter System. In addition to Encounter System functionality, MARS allowed the scanning, viewing, and printing of images, data extractions from forms, and data access through ACUMEN, an internally developed GUI.

By the time of the Davies Award in 1997, MARS was fully implemented in 13 ambulatory care clinics in Cleveland, Ohio, and surrounding communities. Some 220 physicians and 110 allied health professionals used MARS routinely for every patient encounter.

MANAGEMENT

The MARS core team established the following strategic objectives: to improve the quality of care delivered to members, to decrease the organization's operating costs, and to create a stream of data for electronic billing.

Two groups of physicians helped with design and implementation. One provided leadership in the development of ACUMEN, which allowed easy retrieval of results from various information systems. The other, a Physician Advisory Group, addressed areas of system development requiring a consensus opinion among physicians.

While the Encounter System was built internally, the image manipulation part of MARS was a proprietary product of Sequoia Software Corporation called medSTAR. MARS included interfaces to the organization's radiology system, laboratory system (Sunquest), appointment system (medTEC), and membership system (MIPS). Building the system internally brought greater flexibility.

The Ophthalmology Department of the Kaiser facility in Parma, Ohio served as the initial pilot site for MARS. Several approaches were used to gain acceptance. First, the MARS core team took a stepped approach to implementation. The Encounter System, for example, was non-threatening to clinical staff; it provided crucial information without extra work. Second, the team, with complete administrative support, consistently communicated MARS was a staged implementation, not simply a pilot. Team members remained attentive to the emerging needs of the organization. Finally, the MARS team committed to a highly supportive training process. Generous support and coaching assistance were provided for a substantial time period following implementation.

For data and system security, MARS featured password protection and automatic turn off. Off-site access was limited to certain contract hospitals. The project team, in consultation with the mental health and alcohol/chemical dependency departments, the Physician Advisory Group, and in-house legal counsel, developed policies for handling confidential and sensitive information. Security tables were reviewed and modified as new hires, employee transfers, and terminations became effective. All employees signed confidentiality statements.

Following implementation, the MARS project team met regularly with most users in formal and informal settings. The team tracked issues or problems until resolved. A problem analysis center stayed open 24 hours a day, seven days a week.

FUNCTIONALITY

MARS brought a comprehensive database of patient information to Kaiser of Ohio. Initially, the Encounter System captured vital signs, smoking status, diagnoses, medications, allergies, and immunizations. MARS allowed completion of the clinical data set. It captured data elements for preventive healthcare and collected risk information.

MARS' scanning functionality captured data from outside the organization—from hospitalizations prior to enrollment or from outside the Kaiser system. Scanning proved to be the best way for clinicians to receive notes from outside consultants.

A provider-friendly approach to collecting data made MARS very acceptable to clinical staff. Physicians could describe diagnoses in their own words; the system would store both clinical and billing diagnoses. By 1997, a risk assessment form could be printed for any health assessment or physical exam. It collected data relating to unhealthy behaviors, preventive medicine, medical history, and senior citizen functionality.

Anything that was dictated within the organization, or in affiliated hospitals, could be captured and placed in MARS.

All providers had full access. Through ACUMEN, they could review diagnoses, allergies, medications prescribed and dispensed, immunizations, procedures, lab and radiology results, vital signs, status of alerts, reminders, and internal referrals. Providers could access an image file, which included handwritten progress notes, clinical forms, results of procedures, and outside information.

As a decision support tool, MARS proved highly valuable. It generated reminders about clinical guidelines at the point of care. Primary care physicians received quarterly status reports on their success in meeting the guidelines. MARS improved efficiency. Emergency departments and urgent care centers received information previously unavailable, as medical charts were located elsewhere.

MARS supported numerous strategic initiatives involving patient data analysis. Quality goals, such as reductions in mortality from coronary artery disease and reductions in smoking prevalence, were supported by MARS reminders. MARS produced a stream of electronic International Statistical Classification of Diseases and Related Health Problems-9-composite message/composite data type (ICD-9-CM) and Current Procedural Terminology-4 (CPT-4) data to simplify patient accounting.

Data on the number of visits for various types of medical problems was helpful in designing utilization programs. A cost management system was developed using ICD-9-CM/CPT-4 data from MARS. MARS facilitated research, both internal and external. MARS data was crucial to the organization in evaluating outcomes. Finally, the database was useful in evaluating care within Kaiser Permanente of Ohio, compared to other Kaiser regions.

TECHNOLOGY

MARS featured several integrated systems running on two distinct operating environments. The Encounter System collected and processed information related to outpatient visits. The Sunquest Laboratory Information System collected lab orders, tracked orders, and furnished results. The Radiology Information System was developed internally. ACUMEN, a GUI, allowed healthcare providers to view clinical information in a point-and-click fashion. MARS used medSTAR for document processing.

The order entry system served as a central point for placing clinical orders, tracking them, and providing results. Results were delivered to a results queue to be reviewed and approved by the ordering provider. The ACUFIXER System validated information received electronically from external systems—typically, reports and correspondence from community hospitals.

The primary platforms housing these applications were an IBM mainframe and a Microsoft NT distributed computing environment. The IBM environment consisted of a large ES9000 mainframe running the multiple virtual storage (MVS) operating system. The applications ran in a customer information control system (CICS) environment, and used integrated database management system (IDMS), database 2 (DB2), and virtual storage access method (VSAM) to store information. The telecommunications network was a system network architecture (SNA) communicating through T1 lines to 14 facilities.

The client/server environment used to support the imaging application consisted of multiple servers running Microsoft NT Server. Fourteen LANs linked workstations to servers. The LANs were connected via frame relay circuits to make up the WAN. The TCP/IP networking protocol exchanged data between computers.

The MVS mainframe environment used resource access control facility (RACF) security. The NT environment used Microsoft NT's security mechanisms. Both methods required user identifiers and passwords. Access was monitored by security logs noting date, time, user, workstation, and medical record number.

For data integrity, the MVS environment featured tools for managing backup, including scheduling, mirroring, cataloging tapes, and maintaining multiple generations. System integrity was facilitated using redundancies wherever possible.

Kaiser staff worked toward system availability 24 hours a day, seven days a week. Enhancements to the mainframe environment were ongoing, but downtime was necessary one to two hours each night and five hours on Sunday evenings. The client/server environment provided true around the clock availability, except for unplanned outages, which occurred at a rate of less than 1 percent.

VALUE

MARS continued on track to meet the aggressive quality and business goals envisioned by the leaders of Kaiser Permanente of Ohio. Quality of care improved through reliable access to complete patient information. Access extended to external sites, including the Cleveland Clinic, Kaiser's main referral hospital.

MARS generated a growing list of alerts and reminders to support quality initiatives. The reminders addressed preventive health, disease management, and service tracking for referrals and abnormal screening results. Kaiser's smoking cessation program relied heavily on MARS functionality.

The organization received a National Committee for Quality Assurance (NCQA) three-year accreditation. Part of this success stemmed directly from the Encounter System, which fulfilled a requirement for consolidated problem and medication lists at every patient visit.

MARS had a direct impact on clinical outcomes. For example, Kaiser staff sought complete influenza immunization of Medicare patients. MARS supported this effort in several ways. During flu season, reminders were printed as patients were seen. A tape extract of all Medicare-age members, who had not received flu vaccine, triggered an automated telephone device to call patients and suggest a visit. As a result, the overall immunization rate increased by some 12 percent, to a range of 65 to 67 percent. With support from MARS, the rate of child immunizations by age 2 increased to 93 percent, among the best in the country.

The cost of building MARS was approximately $10 million. MARS resulted in annual savings and expenses with net savings of more than $2 million per year. Staff in the medical records department decreased in line with the declining volume of filing paper records and requests for chart pulls. Reminders were used to transition to formulary medications. By providing a stream of data for electronic billing, MARS helped the organization collect revenues it had been unable to collect in the past.

MARS proved to be an excellent research tool. With critical ongoing clinical information on some 200,000 members, MARS supported numerous research studies. Further, MARS facilitated the systematic dispersion of health education and preventive medicine guidelines to an entire population of patients in a cost-effective manner that did not significantly increase the work of clinicians.

For Kaiser Permanente of Ohio, MARS' implementation was a success, bringing benefits system-wide—from improved quality of care, to better communications, cost savings, and greater efficiencies. By 1997, MARS was "at the center of medical care delivery in the organization," and accessed routinely for every patient encounter.

1997 DAVIES ORGANIZATIONAL AWARD WINNER
NORTH MISSISSIPPI HEALTH SERVICES

ABOUT THE ORGANIZATION

North Mississippi Health Services (NMHS) is a non-profit integrated healthcare delivery system serving a population of 600,000 throughout 22 counties in Mississippi, Alabama, and Tennessee. At the time of the Davies Award, the organization owned five hospitals. The largest of these hospitals, and in fact, the largest U.S. hospital in a rural setting, North Mississippi Medical Center, was a 647-bed, tertiary care facility offering 42 medical and surgical specialties.

NMHS sprang from humble beginnings. In 1920, several Tupelo, Mississippi, physicians developed a makeshift hospital in an abandoned YMCA building. After a tornado killed more than 200 people, a 50-bed "Hospital on the Hill" was constructed in 1937.

The hospital grew along with the Tupelo community. In 1961, bed capacity was increased to 200. In 1966, a 100-bed psychiatric unit opened. In 1969, the hospital established a 34-bed satellite facility in Baldwyn, Mississippi, By 1980, the more than 600-bed complex was admitting more than 25,000 patients annually.

In 1982, services and facilities were incorporated under one umbrella, NMHS, as a comprehensive health system. NMHS affiliated with a hospital in West Point, Mississippi, and opened a dialysis center in Oxford, Mississippi. NMHS added a chemical dependency unit, and in 1986, added an outpatient surgical clinic and a dedicated women's hospital.

NMHS' EHR was the result of an integrated planning effort involving leadership from information systems, finance, operations, practicing physicians, and consultants. NMHS took a can-do attitude to go beyond simply developing a link among system components. By working together, NMHS information specialists and clinicians developed a widely accessible EHR that provided patient screening and monitoring tools, along with automated care guides and outcomes analyses.

MANAGEMENT

Building an EHR was challenging for NMHS because of the variety of information demands required by a large health system spread over an extensive rural area. Key to the organization's success was the planning process, led by the Clinical Information System Steering Committee. The committee included leadership from the information system (IS) department, administration, finance, operations, and physicians.

The committee identified four major goals: develop an EHR; provide access to the EHR from any point; assure the system could accommodate managed care; and upgrade technology to enhance communication.

The first step called for an assessment of the NMHS system and an analysis of the NMHS environment. This process identified the components of the clinical system, the ancillary applications, entities supported, and the capabilities of affiliated hospitals.

A review of the network supported the installation of a fiber backbone that connected facilities on the main campus, and a Cabletron Hub-based network for connectivity throughout the system. An assessment of hardware assets brought recommendations for upgrades and more equipment.

As the plan progressed, the IS department staff and budget were increased, with particular emphasis on developing clinical expertise. At the time of the Davies Award, the IS department included 15 registered nurses, a pharmacist, two medical technicians, and a respiratory therapist.

Project teams were formed for the four strategic initiatives. They developed benefits, executed work plans, and were accountable for completion of each project. As implementation progressed, end-user project teams were formed. They outlined policies and procedures, established time frames, adapted services, and devised training programs.

While governance of the information system was provided by the Clinical Information System Steering Committee and individual IS project teams, routine operations were managed by NMHS' multi-disciplinary IS project team. This group met weekly to hear requests for enhancements. Each request was reviewed, examining both its global effect and extended application.

The IS project team also tested new software releases to ensure data integrity and quality. The team routinely checked interfaces to the system to ensure data accuracy, and approved requests for access to specific data elements, voting on each and approving only those that demonstrated true need.

The effectiveness of NMHS' EHR was evaluated in many ways, including routine audits, intermittent user surveys, and external accreditation. After training sessions, user groups provided feedback. Evaluations were carefully reviewed, and feasible suggestions were implemented.

FUNCTIONALITY

The functions of the NMHS EHR evolved over 14 years. Significant data collection, assessment, and feedback dictated additions. At the time of the Davies Award, a survey revealed up to 90 percent of patient information was documented in the automated record.

User concerns were addressed through multiple feedback mechanisms. In addition to broad representation on the IS project team, an IS department office was located in the main hospital, and an IS support technician was available 24 hours per day. Calls from users received immediate attention and clinical analysts made routine rounds on nursing units.

A WAN provided real-time data entry and retrieval. Interfaces allowed for data capture from stand-alone systems located at different points. Dictated reports were transcribed and entered into the patient record. User input facilitated the design of data entry. Over the years, thousands of clinical pathways were developed and customized.

The Cabletron Hub-based network enabled mobile terminals to be used in the emergency department and on patient units. As a result, NMHS' information system was in place at more than 100 different sites in 26 towns in a two-state, 70-mile radius of Tupelo. PCs and printers were available at all NMHS facilities.

With expanded capabilities and more than 4,000 users, access to information became an important confidentiality issue. The IS project team defined information on a need-to-know basis. Each user class had a unique retrieval guide for requesting patient-specific information.

The EHR provided real-time and retrospective clinical decision support, and medical and drug information. The support tools screened patients at risk for adverse events and provided caregivers with individualized clinical information. Care guide critical pathways determined a patient's length of stay and necessary services.

The sheer accessibility of patient information across the integrated system improved efficiency. Lab tests were readily available and did not need to be repeated. Ambulatory care notes could be retrieved by admitting clinicians.

Finally, the EHR was used regularly for administrative and practice management functions. The Center for Business Health and the quality and risk management departments routinely requested data on patient outcomes, charge capture, and resource utilization.

TECHNOLOGY

The NMHS EHR was based on TDS-7000 from Eclipsys Information Services. It ran on an IBM 9121-320 mainframe in a partition controlled by a virtual storage extended/enterprise services architecture (VSE/ESA) operating system. The databases resided on IBM RAMAC-II disk devices attached to the mainframe via enterprise systems connection (ESCON) fiber optic channels. The mainframe communicated with the network using an IBM 3745, model 170, controller that was channel-attached, and interfaced locally with a token ring network. On the token ring were PCs using ADAPTA-SNA software and functioning as gateways to the Ethernet 10-base-T LANs.

Each gateway supported up to 254-user sessions. The LANs connected over a fiber distributed data interface (FDDI) fiber optic backbone. Users communicated with PCs using TDS-7000 software. Tasks were scheduled in priority order: retrieval requests, information updates, and printout generation. Data was entered using a light pen or mouse. Most of the data resided in the patient master file (PMF) of the TDS-7000, where each patient's data was stored by episode of care. An episode was created for each admission. Patient episodes were accessed by name, attending physician, nursing station, patient type, or other. Users could view data across several episodes as a single view.

Security was a top priority. A Security and Confidentiality Committee established two-level sign-on codes, employee agreement documents signed upon hiring, policies for disablement of sign-on codes upon termination, special handling for behavioral patients, and audits of access to patient data.

System and data integrity were critical. TDS-7000 was chosen because of its internal data integrity assurance features. Data entry errors were reduced through input message editing, using forced picks—date of birth required on admission, and route of administration required for medication orders, for example. To address system integrity, a special task force was established with the goal of 100 percent system up time. For power outages, an uninterruptible power supply was installed, first by battery, then by diesel generator. To assure network availability, NMHS moved from a hard point-to-point connection to a standardized network concept [system network architecture/virtual telecommunications access method –Ethernet –Netware (SNA/VTAM—Ethernet—Netware)]. For downtime due to hardware, spare equipment was maintained in strategic areas.

The RAMAC-II disk devices housing the databases featured three ESCON channels attaching the controller to the mainframe. If one channel failed, the others took over. In addition, a disk drawer in the unit was designated the hot spare, a safeguard to database integrity.

VALUE

The EHR provided NMHS opportunities to improve both efficiency and services. In 1988, an adverse drug reaction (ADR) monitoring program was implemented; it relied on the EHR to identify patients at risk. Analysis of the ADRs was the source of several preventive intervention programs, including a pharmacokinetic consult service, and phenytoin and tube feeding screening.

In 1989, software was acquired for monitoring drug-to-drug interactions. Using the EHR, interactions were screened more consistently, up to 25 to 30 per day. An automated drug allergy program was implemented. More than 90 allergies were screened, significantly reducing the number of patients experiencing adverse effects. In 1994, the pharmacy implemented an anticoagulation consult service. It relied on the EHR for information on a patient's coagulation status. The pharmacy also developed a creatinine clearance screening program for which the EHR identified patients requiring pharmacist review and dosage changes.

The EHR provided cumulative data for clinical practice analysis. Resulting modifications brought significant reductions in lengths of stay and lower costs for numerous diagnoses.

NMHS successfully implemented an EHR across its integrated system. Physicians and other caregivers gained access to patient information from anywhere in this geographically extensive system. The end result was better informed and more efficient patient care.

1997 DAVIES ORGANIZATIONAL AWARD WINNER
REGENSTRIEF INSTITUTE FOR HEALTH CARE

ABOUT THE ORGANIZATION

Founded in 1969 by Samuel N. Regenstrief and John B. Hickham, MD, with the mission of studying and improving healthcare, the Regenstrief Institute for Health Care is a privately endowed research organization in Indianapolis. Regenstrief believed the application of systems engineering, industrial engineering, computer science, and statistical techniques could improve the delivery and cost of healthcare.

The Regenstrief Institute represents a collaboration of the Regenstrief Foundation, Indiana University (IU) School of Medicine and its Division of General Internal Medicine, and the Health and Hospital Corporation of Marion County, which operates the Wishard Memorial Hospital. The Regenstrief Institute was the first organization to study computer-based patient record systems in rigorous randomized trials. Its many published studies are well known and heavily cited in the healthcare and information systems communities.

MANAGEMENT

Under the leadership of Clement J. McDonald, MD, then chief of the Computer Science Research Group and now director of the Institute, in 1972, the Regenstrief Institute initiated the Regenstrief Medical Records System (RMRS). The RMRS is a longitudinal, integrated inpatient and outpatient electronic record: its primary goal is to improve patient care while hosting research and education. Its initial aims were as follows: to eliminate the problems associated with the paper record; to deliver information in a more organized and useful way; and to accurately process medical record information and provide decision support to physicians.

At the time the Institute won the Davies Award in 1997, the RMRS contained records for 1.4 million patients and added data from approximately 600,000 ambulatory and 50,000 inpatient encounters per year. The RMRS served four hospitals on the IU Medical Center campus, 40 outpatient clinics and primary care sites, and an extended care facility. Institute investigators and staff involved in RMRS development and application were practicing clinicians in IU's Division of General Internal Medicine, on the medical staff of Wishard Hospital, and on the faculty of medical school. With a culture that encouraged experimentation and frequent feedback from users to identify failures and develop alternative approaches, the Institute coordinated RMRS planning and development.

FUNCTIONALITY

In assessing system needs on the input side, the Regenstrief Institute used the principle of starting with the "lowest-hanging fruit." For example, the RMRS project began by capturing data that was already available in electronic form, such as laboratory data, and only later tackled the capture of structured physician observations during the physical examination and history. On the output side, the goal was to develop programs that would organize, display, and think about the medical record content in useful ways. The project used a rapid prototyping approach that allowed early incorporation of user feedback into system design and development.

The data repository consisted of the Medical Record File, which maintained highly structured and coded observations, and the Text Report Facility, which stored structured and partially coded text. The set of data captured for the record varied at the four hospitals according to each organization's local constraints and realities. For example, outpatient prescriptions could be captured electronically with ease from Wishard Hospital (a county hospital) because most of the hospital's patients obtained their prescriptions at the hospital. The RMRS used electronic interfaces to access data already stored on the four hospitals' other computer systems.

Specially trained technicians encoded free text diagnostic reports, such as cardiac ultrasounds and chest x-rays, in a manner that provided only the impression, rather than all of the information on the narrative report. Because the Institute's staff found physicians more receptive to taking data from the computer rather than providing data to the computer, paper documents at first were the primary means of capturing physicians' observations; other personnel performed the data entry. However, use of workstations for direction capture of physician information began on a large scale as the project progressed.

The RMRS project commenced with physician orders (rather than their notes) because orders had more structure and offered more opportunities for shaping practice patterns through computer feedback. For example, physicians could be provided with feedback about patients at risk for particular problems, the cost consequences of their actions, and ambiguous orders.

The RMRS was accessible to all hospital, clinic, and other care site staff. Decision support was provided through a rule-based reminder system called CARE. Before each scheduled visit, the system reviewed each patient's record according to approximately 600 physician-authored rules, and provided reminders about patient conditions that might need medical attention. Physicians also received decision support for the following: appropriate medications based on medication rules, ideal weight, diet therapy, interventions for patients with high cardiovascular risk, treating under-treated diseases, new abnormalities, and preventive care.

The computer record offered care providers a number of patient visit-associated outputs, which could be viewed either on workstations or on paper. As many as five different reports could be produced for each visit, depending upon the practice's requirements and specifications. The visit encounter form, filled in by the provider and returned to the computer after which some of the data was manually entered, included four sections: the patient's problem list; a list of observation variables, which could be defined by each practice; written notes; and order menus specified by practices not using the clinical workstation to record their orders. The RMRS also could produce summaries of the patient's medical record in abstract and flow sheet form. All of this information could be obtained online via any of the hundreds of terminals placed in the care sites.

RMRS components included an inpatient and outpatient pharmacy system, laboratory system, and various administrative systems, such as an appointment scheduling system. In addition to clinical and administrative applications, the RMRS was used to support research, quality assurance, and other population-based needs.

TECHNOLOGY

Given the number of organizational entities involved in the RMRS, the network infrastructure consisted of a patchwork-like redundant FDDI ring that connected major locations. The central server was a cluster of DEC Virtual Address Extension (VAX) and Alpha computers running the open VMS operating system. The primary clinical data repository and results display applications executed on a high-performance disk array under a relational database developed at the Regenstrief Institute.

The RMRS had a simple but elegant data model with represented objects including patients, providers, locations, institutions, clinical observations, clinical text reports, encounters, surgical procedures, and prescriptions. The RMRS knowledge base was organized by a single, unified concept dictionary, which contained a record for each test, treatment, symptom, finding, diagnosis, measurement unit, and set.

Physical security was assured through controlled access to the servers located in a data center. Physician workstations were in physicians' workrooms and nurses' workstations could be monitored. Data integrity was assured through level 1 redundant array of independent disks (RAID) storage for critical files, level 5 RAID disk storage for less critical files, processor clustering technology, redundant network trunks, and other means. Each user was required to sign an access agreement before being issued an identifier and password. Data exchange standards included HL7, National Council for Prescription Drug Programs (NCPDP), and digital imaging and communications in medicine (DICOM). The system supported multiple communication and networking protocols, but adherence by users to unifying standards was considered extremely important.

VALUE

A user-centric approach to development of the RMRS ensured fast response times and the ability for clinicians to express themselves in a natural way. Its broad user base and long-term existence (more than 25 years in some sites) testify to the system's wide acceptance.

Beginning in the early 1970s, the Institute conducted formal assessments of RMRS user satisfaction, productivity, and effectiveness. Early studies of RMRS use by physicians caring for patients in the emergency department indicated the system's ability to organize and display data substantially reduced testing. In addition, its reminder function increased needed clinical interventions.

For example, the first large-scale study of computer reminders, based on CARE, demonstrated a 20 percent increase in compliance with reminders for all classes of providers, including staff physicians, residents, and nurse practitioners. Reminders focused on needed preventive care, rules suggesting tests needed to identify causes for existing abnormalities and to complete an initial database, messages suggesting prophylactic treatment, and rules about the treatment of active problems, such as guidelines for treating congestive heart failure. The study conclusively showed reminders delivered at the time the physician is delivering care are more effective than those delivered later. Additional studies on use of RMRS clinical workstations to improve the quality of care as judged by compliance with clinical guidelines were underway at the time of the award.

Overall, Regenstrief Institute studies indicated that, to be of value, reminders must be actionable, concise, patient- and task-specific, available at the time of care, constructed to make the task easier, reasonable at least one-third of the time, and appropriate to the available data.

RMRS exemplifies a continuously evolving system in an ever-changing healthcare environment. At the beginning of the RMRS project, the computer system was seen as the goal, and energy was invested in making the best possible system. The clinical data was the incidental grist to the system. The Regenstrief Institute team found reality was the opposite. "All of the work and all of the value are in the data, and the computer system is but a vessel for that data. Systems are replaced every five years; the data stays forever," they noted. The RMRS team concluded as follows: "What has not changed is the commitment of the providers to continuous improvement, and using what works and not necessarily what is appealing. Success lies in implementation, not in technology."

1998 DAVIES ORGANIZATIONAL AWARD WINNER
KAISER PERMANENTE NORTHWEST

ABOUT THE ORGANIZATION

Kaiser Permanente of the Northwest (KPNW) was established as a prepaid healthcare system to serve workers at the Kaiser shipyards in Vancouver, Washington, and in Portland, Oregon, during World War II. With the war's end and the closing of the shipyards in 1945, the organization opened enrollment to the community. Membership increased, and by 1960, KPNW was delivering care at Bess Kaiser Hospital and several outpatient facilities. In 1975, KPNW opened Kaiser Sunnyside Medical Center, and in 1980, expanded its service area to Salem, Oregon. In 1984, the organization opened a medical office in the Longview-Kelso community in Southwest Washington.

In 1996, inpatient utilization declined. KPNW leaders decided to close Bess Kaiser and affiliate with several community hospitals. At the time of the Davies Award, KPNW provided care to more than 400,000 capitated members at Kaiser Sunnyside Medical Center, six community hospitals, and 21 medical offices.

KPNW's CIS was both a comprehensive EHR and a system that automated the information transmission processes related to outpatient care. More than 700 physicians and clinicians, representing more than 20 medical and surgical specialties, and 2,600 support staff in 27 geographically separate sites, used the CIS to deliver care.

MANAGEMENT

In 1990, KPNW established a governance process for information services, led by an Information Services Steering Committee. This committee developed strategic plans, capital budgets, and policies for information services. In 1993, Northwest Permanente hired an assistant medical director for clinical systems—a move to encourage the swift development and implementation of an EHR.

In 1991, work began to develop a results reporting system (RRS), a read-only repository of clinical data derived from ancillary systems. RRS data merged electronically accessible and clinically relevant data into a single patient-centered database that included demographic and benefits information, outpatient pharmacy data, dictated reports, laboratory data, tumor registry data, and inpatient admission, discharge, and transfer (ADT) data.

RRS clearly demonstrated the power of computer technology to improve a clinician's ability to provide medical care. Its success paved the way for clinicians' acceptance of EpicCare, a more comprehensive component of the EHR. EpicCare automated all outpatient documentation, ordering and messaging processes.

In 1993, a pilot phase of EpicCare commenced, and by 1994, EpicCare was in use by 46 primary care clinicians in two outpatient medical offices. User surveys found clinician attitudes to be increasingly positive as proficiency developed. The system was technically adequate, flexible, and easy to modify. By 1996, full deployment was underway and by year-end 1997, some 700 clinicians used EpicCare as their core documentation and communications tool.

Multimedia computer-based interactive training was the primary teaching tool for EpicCare. Learners had the freedom to train at their own pace and schedules. Interactive training was augmented by paper and Web-based documents, classroom sessions, and individual and go-live support.

From the start, clinicians found diagnosis code selection to be difficult. The project team examined codes used by three comparable organizations. This analysis eliminated some obscure and infrequently used codes and consolidated others. A verbatim utility was added to allow clinicians to modify a textual description to suit an exact need.

KPNW had a long history of protecting patient confidentiality. EHR safeguards included:

• Individual accounts, passwords, and policies prohibiting sharing;
• Signed confidentiality statements;
• Detailed logs of all read and write activity;
• Routine review of suspected breaches by the Confidentiality Committee;
• Restrictions on users, based on position;
• Sequestration of sensitive information;
• Protection of the record against changes following a patient encounter;
• Time-outs; and
• Policies to report and track potential breaches.

FUNCTIONALITY

KPNW's RRS required little effort from clinicians. The system featured a consistent user interface, using a single keystroke navigation scheme. It was patient centric, allowing for summary and detailed views of data, and the ability to scan a chart to view information.

In the outpatient setting, providers used EpicCare to document, order, refer, and message. Guidelines and medication suggestions were provided in-line to clinicians. Buttons along the top and bottom of the screen allowed access to various capabilities: reviewing the chart, charting, ordering, and prescribing.

Data captured by EpicCare was comprehensive, incorporating both coded discreet data and narrative information. Diagnoses, problem lists, past history, medication lists, orders, results, reasons for visits, telephone encounters, immunization records, allergies, and smoking status could be found in EpicCare.

Most user entry required keyboarding, with a dictation option for the subjective and objective portion of encounters. Keyboard entry was facilitated through field defaults, selection lists, string-matching, and synonym matching. System templates, boilerplate text with fill-in-the-blank areas, and drop-down pick lists could be retrieved with two key strokes. Each department developed its own smart-text templates and system phrases. Clinicians had their own phrase lists.

Both RRS and EpicCare were widely available. All clinicians had dedicated workstations, as did clinic assistants, advice nurses, triage and treatment room nurses, and personnel in laboratory, radiology and pharmacy. RRS and EpicCare were available in allied hospitals. All users were assigned to a security class that defined the functions and data they could access. Some were restricted to review function only; others could access review, ordering, and prescribing functions. EpicCare enforced cosignatures for users such as residents and advice nurses.

Decision support features were numerous. Paper summaries allowed clinicians to review recent tests and immunizations before office visits. Guidelines could be embedded into the order entry pathway. Clinicians ordering prescriptions that were not on the formulary received messages suggesting alternatives. SmartRx provided guidance on recommended medications. Online guidelines advised clinicians on how and when to refer patients to specialists.

SmartSets supported best-care decisions by bringing together diagnoses, lab and imaging orders, medication and procedure orders, and patient information and supporting documentation to a single tailored screen. EpicCare included extensive messaging functions.

KPNW evaluated the EHR system often and published its findings. Clinicians immediately embraced RRS. By March 1994, users were accessing 11,450 information screens daily. The EpicCare rollout, by contrast, was gradual. Still, by November 1996, 736 clinicians, 1,317 clinical staff, and 801 others were regular users. A survey from early 1997 found 63 percent of respondents agreeing with the statement, "EpicCare is worth the time and effort to use it."

TECHNOLOGY

The KPNW RRS ran on DEC VAX 7620 using the VMS operating system and record management services (RMS) file structure. All files were shadowed; internal CPU hardware was redundant. The RRS was available over an Ethernet-based area wide routed network connected to the internal network via TCP/IP, local area transport (LAT), and Digital Equipment Corporation Network (DECnet).

The EpicCare medical record application was a client/server system developed by Epic Systems. EpicCare's GUI was written in Microsoft Visual Basic and ran on Intel-based PC workstations. KPNW's implementation of EpicCare used Intersystem's ANSI-M proprietary database management system. Workstations were networked into one Windows NT domain served by dual NT servers in each clinic. EpicCare's database server was a Digital Alpha 8440-10.

The RRS user interface featured a character cell-based application developed using DEC's FMS COBOL. EpicCare was a client/server application that separated the visual basic (VB) front end from the ANSI-M database back end, allowing for easy modification and user interface functionality. RRS maintained data from multiple sources reformatted and indexed by patient. The system received data loads from all clinical systems. Though nightly loads were most common, some happened every 15 minutes. EpicCare transmitted data from outside sources in real time.

The IS department monitored storage needs, adding disk space, as needed. Both hardware and software could be added in a plug-and-play manner. Any number of processors, plus memory and disk storage, could be added without changing the system. The KPNW EHR complied with organizational security requirements. Patient-specific data from EpicCare and RRS resided on database servers physically located in

Kaiser's data center. Physical access was restricted. All RRS data was shadowed, and the system featured weekly full-image and nightly incremental backups. Two levels of disk shadowing, RAID 5 technology, nightly backups, and M journaling ensured EpicCare's database integrity.

RRS was available wherever there was a virtual terminal (VT) and a modem or network connection. RRS could be accessed by clinicians from home, at allied hospitals, or in medical offices. EpicCare was available 24 hours per day, except for 25 minutes nightly for system updates and backup. For data integrity and confidentiality, all RRS and EpicCare activity was logged in detail. The logs were invaluable for researching confidentiality incidents. Three mirrored databases and RAID 5 striping provided an extreme measure of data redundancy and safety.

VALUE

KPNW's EHR coincided with unprecedented change and upheaval for clinicians. The organization relied on dialog and feedback, plus objective measurement, to guide continued development. Respondents to a 1997 survey overwhelmingly agreed EpicCare improved the legibility and availability of chart notes. EpicCare improved documentation of patient conditions and supported disease-based population care.

The EHR produced a comprehensive medical record at any time and any location. Of 423 clinicians surveyed in 1997, more than half thought EpicCare and RRS contributed to better telephone advice. Focus groups identified the following as improving efficiencies system-wide: RRS summaries, online displays of patient encounters, online clinician schedules, and SmartRxs.

The EHR decreased the costs of care by preventing unnecessary tests and identifying less costly options, and reduced clinician phone calls to the laboratory for results. Outpatient lab tests per enrolled member declined, thanks to an improved ability to access existing results. The medical records department eliminated three positions responsible for ad hoc chart pulls. EpicCare supported formulary drug prescribing by providing online prompts. Quick access to patient information, allowing for timely identification of health issues, often by phone, brought a decrease in visits per member annually.

The impact of an EHR on an organization the size and complexity of KPNW was multifaceted and pervasive. RRS and EpicCare integrated the delivery of care for KPNW's 400,000 members. Clinicians received instant access to a comprehensive EHR to enter and retrieve information on any member in any of 27 different settings. Seamless decision support guided best practices and reduced unnecessary variations. Equally significant, EpicCare allowed the organization to capture clinical data for business needs, outcomes analysis, and research.

1998 DAVIES ORGANIZATIONAL AWARD WINNER
NORTHWESTERN MEMORIAL HOSPITAL

ABOUT THE ORGANIZATION

Located in the heart of downtown Chicago's Gold Coast, Northwestern Memorial Hospital (NMH) is a 700-bed private, not-for-profit academic medical center. NMH was formed through the 1972 merger of Passavant and Wesley Hospitals, whose histories date back to as early as the 1880s. It serves as the primary teaching hospital of Northwestern University Medical School. At the time NMH won the Davies Award, the hospital had approximately 1,200 physicians and more than 4,000 nursing and other employees who provided patient care during 36,000 inpatient admissions and 50,000 outpatient visits.

In 1993, five years prior to the award, NMH's umbrella organization—Northwestern Memorial Corporation—made a long-range commitment to clinical integration and named CIS as an essential infrastructure for the organization's healthcare delivery environment. The parent organization embarked on an initiative to implement a state-of-the-art CIS to support its tripartite mission of patient care, research, and education.

Concurrent with this initiative, NMH successfully obtained a $3.1 million research contract sponsored by the National Library of Medicine to conduct a CIS demonstration project. Titled NetReach, the project studied the information needs of clinicians, acquired and developed information tools to address the needs, and introduced a computer-based patient record (EHR) system as a new foundation for managing clinical information. The NetReach Project involved seven different clinical sites in order to reflect the diversity of physician practices on Northwestern's campus.

MANAGEMENT

NMH established the following vision for its CIS: "To continuously evolve a state-of-the-art CIS that enhances the efficiency and effectiveness of healthcare teams by providing relevant information anywhere, any time in support of patient care, management research, and education."

NMH's medical staff is a mixture of community and academic primary care and specialty care physicians. Due to the effect the diversity of practices could have on clinical information needs and the tools necessary to meet the needs, the NetReach project commenced with a comprehensive assessment of user information needs. Surveys, interviews, and various other types of studies were conducted, but observational studies—capable of gleaning information on actual physician information practices—provided the most valuable data. To obtain such information, a team of clinical consultants shadowed physicians at seven different practice sites.

Needs assessment data indicated NMH's clinicians had five high-level information needs: integrated access to patient information; ready access to summary information (for example, problem lists, medications, and demographics); timely and efficient communication among healthcare team members; effective means of providing patient instructions and education; and convenient access to computer work stations with good training and technical support.

The project team produced a list of functional requirements to address these needs, and explored existing clinical patient record (EHR) products and the possibility of developing applications internally. Evaluation criteria included availability of appropriate commercial products, internal development capabilities, project timeline, and budgetary constraints.

The team selected EpicCare®, an EHR system developed by Epic Systems of Madison, Wisconsin, and implemented the EHR system at two pilot sites—a faculty practice and an independent private practice, both with internal medicine physicians. Due to the interest in applying the technology hospital-wide, as appropriate, the NetReach project studied the impact of using an EHR in a controlled environment. Approximately half of the clinicians in the pilot sites used an EHR (participants were called piloteers) and the remainder used traditional paper records.

Staff resources for the project included the clinical consultant team, which was responsible for front-line liaison with the clinician users, and a technical team, which was responsible for hardware, networking, software installation, and system operation. At the time, only a few of the piloteers had computers in their homes or office. The implementation process thus involved considerable change or cultural management to acclimatize all participants to the computer as an integral tool for their daily professional lives, for access to information resources, and for clinical patient record system use and management.

Prior to the go-live date (summer 2006), the teams obtained detailed information from physicians to develop lists used in the EHR, such as common encounter diagnoses, reasons for visit, common medications (including default instructions), frequently used medical and surgical history diagnoses and procedures, and other critical information. Formal training on the EHR system began four weeks before the go-live date. The project, in fact, established continuous development and training as the operative standard, using "pizza-induced piloteer meetings" to solicit feedback, share user tips, and provide training with new functionality. The team provided 24/7 user support to the pilot sites.

FUNCTIONALITY

Outpatient data stored in the EHR included demographics, schedules, progress notes, lab test results, and radiology reports. The stored inpatient data included demographics, lab test results, radiology reports, discharge summaries, operative reports, pathology reports, dictated history & physicals (H&Ps), and electrocardiogram (ECG) interpretations.

Major EHR system functionality included the following:
• Chart review addressed the need identified through the assessment process for an integrated view of patient data and included data from encounters, referrals,

procedures, test results, health histories, problem lists, and health maintenance records.

- Patient SnapShot addressed the need for quick access to summary information by providing a summary view of a patient's problem list, medications, allergies, alerts, and other important items.
- Charting tools documented histories, vital signs, physical exams, and progress notes.
- Patient histories included problems, family history, social history, and other histories.
- In basket addressed the need for integrated communications by linking all communications in EpicCare to a patient chart.
- Health maintenance rules identified when clinicians should issue patients reminders about needed preventive interventions.
- Order entry automatically included in the progress note all test and medication orders.
- Drug interactions warned clinicians of potential drug-allergy, drug-food, and drug-drug conflicts.
- Patient education and instructions printed an after-visit summary at the end of a patient encounter.

With the integral participation of clinicians, the team also developed rules-based decision support functionality. Through this functionality and the capabilities identified above, the EHR provided the information framework for continuously improving patient care and managing healthcare delivery.

TECHNOLOGY

Given the goal of providing clinicians with access to patient information anywhere and any time, the team deployed workstations in all of the common settings where physicians access patient records, including clinic exam rooms, clinic nursing stations, the hospital, home, and administrative offices.

The Epic system EHR architecture employed a split logic model in which the application logic was split between the client and the server. The seven NetReach clinical sites were all connected to NMH's fiber optic backbone via T1 connections or better. Using the HL7 standard for messaging, the EHR software was highly scalable and designed to be mission-critical by having redundant CPUs and disk arrays to enhance availability. Backup was designed to occur nightly and did not require the system to be down. Disaster recovery plans were in place.

The EHR system preserved the privacy of patient data through confidentiality policies and application security, which was controlled at multiple levels. Access outside the network was controlled through a password-protected system. The technology and standards provided ubiquitous secure access to patient data for participating NMH clinicians.

VALUE

NMH's NetReach project defined the ultimate measure of an EHR to be its return on information. Whether in support of individual patient care or population health improvement, the hospital expected an EHR system to provide an accessible repository of clinical data and management information tools. The project team defined and measured the EHR's return on information in multiple realms, including the following:

- **Availability and completeness of the patient record**- Complete and available encounter documentation was present in the EHR sooner than in the paper chart. On average, clinicians required 1.3 days to initiate and close EHR patient encounter documentation and 5.2 days for a paper record. The ability to find information in the patient record was and is critical to appropriate and timely patient care.
- **Continuous quality improvement**- Produced as a by-product of patient care, the clinical database of an EHR system was recognized by the team as an evolving store of aggregate patient data. Analyses of data provided powerful tools for continuous quality improvement, quality management, clinical research, fulfillment of reporting requirements, and process improvement.
- **Improving compliance with clinicians' intentions**- The team found use of an EHR's decision support functionality significantly increased clinicians' compliance with their own intentions, such as consistent use of clinical guidelines for influenza vaccination, treatment of moderate or severe asthma with inhaled corticosteroids, and treatment of congestive heart failure (CHF) with angiotensin converting enzyme (ACE) inhibitor therapy. Prior to implementation of the EHR, for example, clinicians clearly endorsed influenza vaccination, but their actual vaccination rates averaged 39 percent. With EHR-based computerized reminders, the EHR users increased their immunization rates 77 percent over their baseline rates to 68 percent, while the control group did not significantly change (from 28 percent to 30 percent).
- **Disease management**- Analysis of patient populations possible through EHR data aggregation enabled NMH staff to identify patients who should be enrolled in disease management programs.
- **Use of the EHR to facilitate clinical research**- Coupling the day-to-day observations in clinical practice with the aggregate data in the online database, the team noted a potentially significant change in the antibiotic-susceptibility of an organism responsible for a common infection. NMH recognized the EHR as an efficient tool for facilitating the discovery of other new knowledge.
- **User satisfaction**- The perceived value of the EHR system by clinicians and its effect on their patient care, obtained via a questionnaire instrument at multiple points, indicated providers using an EHR felt they were better able to manage patient records, make more informed decisions that improved patients' clinical outcomes, and practice more cost effectively.
- **Patient satisfaction**- Use of an EHR also increased the satisfaction of patients, who received a printout that included tailored instructions at the end of every visit.

NMH's NetReach team concluded as follows: "Using a computer-based patient record is essential to providing continuously improving quality healthcare to the population we serve. Above all, it satisfies the mission of our health system: to be an academic medical center where the patient comes first."

EVOLUTION OF THE HOSPITAL'S EHR TO-DATE
AND LESSONS TO SHARE

Challenges Addressed

In the years following the NetReach project, NMH faced and addressed numerous challenges. The first challenge was many physicians were not facile with computers. One tactic that worked for the hospital was introducing e-mail and other basic functionalities to physicians during the year prior to the go-live date. This successfully encouraged physicians to become more computer savvy.

The second challenge was there was limited information available electronically. The hospital traditionally had available basic laboratory, microbiology, and x-ray reports. However, nuclear medicine reports, echo, neuro-testing, and other information was on a different server and not available. Despite some difficulties, NMH did successfully roll out the Epic system to its primary care general internists and, through a controlled experiment funded by the National Library of Medicine, documented a large number of improvements resulting from system use.

The third challenge involved continuing to roll out the EHR during a period of significant demands on the organization, including the building of the new hospital, which opened in 1999. As a result of competing demands, the hospital-based EHR rollout was deferred and the full-time faculty group practice was encouraged to proceed with continued roll out. Working collaboratively with the Faculty Foundation, NMH successfully transitioned to a licensing agreement with Epic and, in late 1999 through 2000, the Faculty Foundation began to expand the EHR throughout the practice's other specialties.

Once the licensing agreement was fully in effect for the Faculty Foundation, challenges included engaging certain specialty physicians and surgical departments, which had highly varied EHR needs and interests. Some subspecialists with very unique needs required customized templates, and in some cases new interfaces to additional technology. A number of surgical specialists, who worked closely with nurse practitioners, required design flexibility for new electronic and work flow solutions.

Lessons to Be Shared

The NetReach project provided numerous value-related lessons that helped to further EHR use organization-wide at Northwestern Memorial Hospital. The key lesson cited by leaders is the classic Pareto's Principle, also known as the 80/20 Rule, which encourages leaders to focus on the 20 percent that really matters.

At NMH, this involved getting a department started with their most important requests related to the EHR but not waiting until every detail was worked out to implement the EHR. Careful planning and development of common order sets, frequently used default medication profiles, and required templates are key before rollout, but NMH advises other organizations not to wait until every single request is answered. An optimization plan, which involves circling back by planners and implementers after six months to review progress, is also very helpful.

Other strategies or tips offered by NMH include the following:

- Spend a modest amount of time instructing physicians about how to relate to patients when they are using an EHR in the exam room. Some principles of physician-patient communication are in order, particularly the importance of sharing the record with patients in the exam room so the EHR is not perceived as a barrier to the physician-patient relationship. Patients generally appreciate the rapid availability of information and understand how the EHR can enhance the quality of their care.

- If implementing an EHR throughout a large practice with multiple departments, start with those departments likely to be most successful. Again, some flexibility with work flow and how the EHR is used should be provided in order to roll out these types of changes in a large organization.

- In justifying the expense of an EHR in NMH's group practice, it was helpful to cite even a modest improvement in reimbursement resulting from the increased ease of documentation for services provided and other charge capture. A reimbursement increase on the order of 4 percent was sufficient ROI to help justify the initial outlay.

- Involve administrative and nursing staff in addition to physicians in the group.

- When identifying and implementing reminders, limit reminders to a small subset with the highest possible value. This is achieved by looking at absolute impact per patient. Although physician reminders are of critical value, alert fatigue is common. A balance should be reached with requests and potential reminders due to the numbing effect they can have on physicians in a busy practice.

- Increase the specificity of reminders. Practitioners should not be inappropriately reminded to do something for a patient who on the surface would appear to qualify for a certain procedure or treatment, but based on the inclusion of a bit of additional knowledge available in the EHR would not be eligible.

The EHR Today

EHR implementation by NMH has continued to positively and significantly enhance the organization's provision of healthcare, particularly related to the quality of documentation, quality of care delivery, and patient safety. Many of these results have been published in the healthcare literature.

In terms of specifics, the organization uses practice alerts to achieve extremely high levels of compliance with comprehensive preventive strategies for healthy patients, such as pap smears, mammograms, and colon cancer screening, and comprehensive treatment strategies for patients with chronic conditions, such as diabetes, congestive heart failure, and asthma.

The organization recently implemented comprehensive individual physician feedback reports on diabetes care, which position the organization well for the new pay-for-performance era.

In 2007, the electronic health record is fully deployed in all respects at Northwestern Memorial Hospital. EHR-based problem lists, medications, physician order entry, and documentation are used by virtually all of the organization's 550-member physician group practice. There are thousands of users within the Faculty Foundation, including many hundreds of house staff physicians. The final departments about to go live on Epic include ophthalmology and psychiatry.

1999 DAVIES ORGANIZATIONAL AWARD WINNER
KAISER PERMANENTE COLORADO REGION

ABOUT THE ORGANIZATION

In 1991, leaders of the Kaiser Permanente Colorado Region, which cares for 350,000 members, initiated a large-scale project with relatively simple, but far-reaching goals. They sought to design and implement a comprehensive ambulatory care CIS for clinicians and members that improved medical care by: making patient information available to caregivers at any time or location without chart lockout; creating a central repository of clinical data for examination of relationships between interventions and outcomes; automating care processes to improve efficiency and reduce costs; and providing effective methods of clinical decision support to positively influence medical decision-making.

The Kaiser Permanente Colorado Region enjoyed a long tradition of partnership between the Kaiser Foundation Health Plan and the Colorado Permanente Medical Group (CPMG). Managers on both sides were accountable for the success of the enterprise. Both groups contributed personnel and resources.

By 1998, CIS implementation sites included 25 facilities: 15 medical offices, four mental health offices, three administrative offices, one emergency department, and two hospitals. The total user population included approximately 500 physicians, 2,000 health plan staff, and 100 medical students/resident physicians.

MANAGEMENT

During the early 1990s, leaders of Kaiser Foundation Health Plan and CPMG asked the information/strategic services department (ISD), CPMG, and clinic operations to predict how clinical computing would best meet healthcare needs in the dynamic marketplace of the future. A Resource Committee, consisting of 12 members from the medical group, and eight from clinic operations and ISD, defined strategic objectives and clarified early requirements of what would become CIS.

Over the course of 1991, the Resource Committee researched existing systems and developed an initial set of functional requirements. Kaiser Permanente Colorado Region and IBM signed a fixed price contract to cover the work.

Representatives of every clinical and administrative department that interacted with the medical record were interviewed regarding their use of the record, their perceived needs for an EHR, business and patient work flow, and current capabilities. Requirements were prioritized.

Clinical, business, IT, and vendor experts developed project timelines, continuously monitoring progress and updating plans. End users were broadly represented during requirements definition, design, development, test, and implementation phases; their input guided changes.

Due to the size and complexity of the implementation and the broad range of user skills, implementation was divided into two phases:

1. Limited access involved installation and stabilization of all hardware/software/ networks and user training focused on read-only capability and customization functions, and

2. Full access involved training in all remaining chart update functions, ordering, processing, and baselets. Baselets were preconfigured, stored views of information concepts and objects taken from the lexicon to speed note entry and other provider functions.

By December 15, 1997, approximately 2,500 users had completed limited access training. Full access rollout for the remainder of the local market began April 1, 1998.

As each medical office or department began full access training, they embarked upon an eight-week boot camp. The first four weeks taught clinicians how to document progress notes on CIS. Electronic ordering was added early; coded assessments followed. The final stage incorporated the use of coded baselets.

CIS' primary design features to support data integrity, timeliness, and reliability rested on the controlled medical terminology (CMT) and the lexicon. System architecture and the deployment of workstations in all areas—offices, exam rooms, nursing stations—allowed for real-time data capture, and communication between CIS and ancillary systems, as well as simultaneous multiple user access to the same chart data. Redundancy, replication, and high availability features, backup/restore and disaster recovery processes ensured the integrity of the patient chart.

Executive support for CIS was clear, visible, and consistent throughout the life of the project.

FUNCTIONALITY

CIS centered on the patient, but its design supported clinical teams in communicating information and managing duties—informing, validating, signing, authenticating, and reviewing—that occurred across patients in the in basket.

Authorized users could pull records in a number of forms, including fact-sheet, stat chart, and complete chart. Individual orders or result or note objects could be accessed from the in basket. Over 1 million charts were available to users.

Workstations were located in offices, exam rooms, nursing quads, and several administrative locations. Users could access CIS 24 hours a day, seven days a week. CIS supported concurrent use of multiple or single records by multiple or single providers without lockout; all computers were available to any authorized user.

Ancillary services were interfaced via HL7 for fully automated linked order entry, results reporting, and automatic documentation.

Chart viewing was flexible, with drill down—summary/detail/prior order— navigation in any direction vertically or horizontally, maintaining the look and feel of the familiar medical record. Advanced views and navigation capabilities were built in for more advanced users, including full keyboard rather than mouse operation.

Charting was carried out through point-and-click and occasional typing. Voice capture/transcription and drawing capability, plus support for scanned, video, and audio images, were present.

Lists of organized but individually modifiable terms were drawn from the lexicon to facilitate coded data entry. Called custom formularies, these lists included diagnoses laboratory and imaging procedures, and clinical findings. Users could maintain the own formularies modified for individual use. They could assign nicknames withc altering the related, unique Systematized Nomenclature of Medicine (SNOMED) codes, facilitating rapid data entry. Since the majority of information entered into the record was derived from these formularies, the data had a high degree of accuracy.

Baselets, as defined earlier, came from an accepted enterprise library, but could be altered and stored in personal files by users. Different users handled baselets in different ways, a majority preferring to use shorter baselets—called baselet fragments—for greater flexibility in clinical situations. By 1998, approximately 53,000 personal baselets were in use.

TECHNOLOGY

The Kaiser Permanente Colorado Region CIS addressed two key functional requirements: maintaining a complete electronic patient record, and automating key clinical processes. The application achieved these goals by integrating into, instead of replacing, departmental systems.

The CIS featured three types of external interfaces, with support for each encapsulated in a separate subsystem:
• A GUI provided all user interface functions.
• A CMT Interface included the functions necessary to interface with the CMT knowledge base.
• An ancillary interface incorporated functions required to interface with external systems.

The CIS supported, but did not require, the distribution of data across multiple physical systems. All of the data management subsystems executed on the UNIX platform and used an underlying relational database management system (RDBMS).

Before accessing the system, a log-on process requiring a personal password authenticated all CIS users. To support healthcare teams, CIS provided a lock-up and transfer capability. Each chart entry was assigned a confidentiality level. The CIS maintained an audit log of all transactions.

The CIS ensured data integrity through the RDBMS for persistent storage. Replication ensured a patient's record could be accessed in read-only mode in the event of system failure. Entries were never deleted.

All data exchanges with external systems used HL7-conforming protocols. Most of the data maintained by the CIS was codified. All network communications used the TCP/IP protocol.

The CIS supported a multi-tier client/server configuration. CIS architecture was scalable across multiple servers and database instances to support nearly any size medical group.

The CIS featured integral support for remote system management and software fault tolerance coupled with a high-availability hardware and network configuration to ensure continuous availability of critical data.

CIS was configured for on-the-fly data backups. Critical patient and provider data replicated from master databases to slave databases in real time, providing another level of backup.

Project leaders monitored system and user performance regularly. A 24/7 command center augmented by multi-site manual monitoring provided system administration and support.

VALUE

CIS project leaders estimated initial financial gains to operations at $3.39 million. The most notable cost savings included reduced dictation for specialties in which physicians substituted baselets, diminished numbers of non-appointment paper chart retrievals, and operational efficiencies in ancillary departments.

Patient records were available at the patient's home clinic, as well as remote clinics, urgent care centers, emergency departments, hospitals, and advice/call centers 24 hours a day. This real-time access to current data streamlined decision-making and rapidity of treatment. Desktop medicine performed via the CIS in basket allowed patient information to be accessed from all sites by any authorized user, facilitating continuity of care and greatly improving inter-clinician communication.

Prescriptions pre-entered with the appropriate dose, dosing interval, and patient instructions decreased risk of medication errors. The CIS automated laboratory and radiology order entry-results review, allowing clinicians to track patients more satisfactorily. Baselets supported guidelines for diagnosis, investigation, and treatment with built-in reminders.

Clinicians enthusiastically embraced CIS as they understood the impact of clinical decision support features on their ability to provide higher quality patient care. In CIS, decision support was present in five distinct ways:
- Information availability at the time of decision-making;
- Guideline-based instructions presented in real time;
- Formulary use that standardized care;
- Baselet use containing integrated documentation/intervention reminders; and
- Intranet access to protocols, guidelines, and utilization data.

Colorado Kaiser leaders concluded, "We believe that the trials and tribulations of developing and implementing a system this comprehensive and this integrated were worthwhile on almost every level. We anticipate new challenges in mastering, mining, and harvesting gains from the enormous amount of data CIS generates, and are hopeful the results of such analysis can be used to help clinicians and their patients make better decisions about medical care."

1999 DAVIES ORGANIZATIONAL AWARD WINNER
THE QUEEN'S MEDICAL CENTER

ABOUT THE ORGANIZATION

When The Queen's Medical Center (QMC or Queen's) received the Davies Award in 1999, it was the largest tertiary care community hospital in Hawaii. With 1,200 affiliated physicians, QMC served as the cornerstone of The Queen's Health System, which also owned and operated 12 ambulatory care clinics—seven clinics with a total of 30 physicians on the island of Oahu and another five clinics with 22 physicians on Maui and Hawaii. At the time, the main campus of QMC included two physicians' office buildings that housed 237 affiliated physicians. In addition, the health system provided home care services on Oahu, Maui, and Hawaii.

Through its EHR initiative, Advanced Clinical Information System (ACIS), The Queen's Medical Center sought to align patients, clinicians, and payors in a process that improved healthcare across the spectrum of patient needs. To do so required not just changes in practice, but a substantial investment in information and performance improvement to achieve better clinical decisions and processes. During the first three years, a critical mass of clinician use and functionality resulted in added value through better decision-making, improved quality and cost outcomes, and a substantial ROI.

Successes achieved included improvements to patient care in many measurable, marketable, and significant ways. In the long run, however, the organizational lessons learned—including listening, planning, and project management that unified clinical practice, process, and information technology—may have proved most beneficial.

MANAGEMENT

In 1993, the specter of healthcare reform and managed care was the driving force for developing an ACIS at Queen's. The survival of Queen's depended upon building a seamless integrated healthcare delivery system. A Clinical Information System Steering Committee—including physician, nursing, and administrative leadership—was formed to develop a computer-based ACIS at the point of care that would substantially improve clinical decision-making.

Early on, the committee established two important philosophical positions: greater benefit would come from supporting better clinical decisions and processes than from simply computerizing existing care patterns, and physicians, as the principal decision makers regarding patient care, must use ACIS.

The Queen's Clinical Performance Improvement model began with an operational acute patient management system that captured critical patient information. Called CLiQ, Clinical Information at Queen's, the system developed was an acute care, physician-oriented, order entry, results reporting system, the Eclipsys 7000. This operational patient management system included an interface engine (STC Datagate) that linked CLiQ to legacy systems, the short message service (SMS) ADT system, and information systems from the laboratory, imaging, pathology, pharmacy, patient accounting, and medical records departments. MedicaLogic, an ambulatory care system, and PtCT Home Care, were added later.

To implement CLiQ and obtain widespread physician use from the start required a critical mass of clinically relevant data. Queen's chose to implement CLiQ rapidly throughout the inpatient units over an 18-month period. For six weeks, a pilot project on two nursing units resolved operational and system problems. Activating the remainder of the hospital took place over the following eight weeks. As each unit was started, CLiQ support staff stayed on the unit 24 hours a day for two weeks to assist physicians and nurses. More than 40,000 hours of training were required to educate more than 2,900 people.

Queen's achieved widespread physician use through a multi-part strategy that included a Physicians Clinical Informatics Group (PCIG), personal order sets, departmental order sets, a Maximum Physician Use Strategy adopted by the Medical Executive Committee, and extensive physician support.

The ability to customize screens and order pathways was critical to implementing CLiQ successfully. Customizing screens for specialties and departments provided an excellent opportunity to engage and involve a large number of users, creating a sense of ownership.

Within a few months, Queen's developed a population management system called the Enterprise Data Warehouse (EDW), an Oracle database that captured all clinical transactions from CLiQ and related systems. The purpose of the EDW was to enable clinicians to manage specific patient populations based on detailed analysis of the process and outcomes of care.

User surveys, electronic messages incorporated into the CLiQ system, monthly meetings of the Medical Informatics Subcommittee, a paid medical director for clinical informatics, and a highly responsive CLiQ staff kept Queen's informed about user needs and satisfaction. Complaints about CLiQ received prompt attention.

Success required the whole medical center be informed and engaged. Constant communication in the form of newsletters, electronic messages, monthly meetings, quality sessions, and presentations was essential to creating an information and improvement culture within Queen's.

"We have shifted away from opinion-based decision-making toward data-based decision-making with ACIS. What was once considered a threat is now perceived as an important tool for clinical performance improvement by evidence-based outcomes," said the CLiQ leadership team.

FUNCTIONALITY

Keeping quality patient care as its primary concern, Queen's designed the components of its EHR to support all individuals involved in delivering patient care. By understanding how patients flow through and interact with the care delivery system, Queen's was able to identify clinical and non-clinical user classes for which the EHR enhanced the care process. Each user class had detailed and specific parameters that defined user access and function.

The Queen's EHR initiative began in the acute care setting with the Eclipsys 7000 (CLiQ) and EDW as initial applications. CLiQ captured and managed order entry, order management, results from major ancillary services, vital signs, intake and output, medication administration, and other documentation. CLiQ allowed patient data to be viewed in single or multiple episode contexts.

Data entry in CLiQ was primarily through point-and-click mouse or light-pen interface; typing was minimized through extensive menus and pre-packaged order sets. CLiQ was widely available on more than 400 workstations throughout the Queen's campus, in the local physicians' office buildings, and in central Honolulu. Clinical workstations were given access to the MicroMedex drug database. In addition, one CLiQ workstation on each nursing unit was designated as a CLiQ Plus Workstation that included access to additional electronic knowledge bases, literature searching, and the Hawaii Medical Library.

CLiQ provided immediate electronic communication of all orders to nursing units and ancillary departments. For laboratory, imaging, and pharmacy, orders interfaced directly into departmental systems. Statim (STAT) medication orders were sent directly to a nurse's alphanumeric pager. Summary reports, such as the CLiQ Quick Scan, were used online and in paper form by nurses, medical staff, and residents for communication with one another. Reporting capability also supported shift-to-shift reporting and hands-off to external agencies.

Clinician satisfaction with CLiQ remained high from its initial activation in 1995. At the time of the Davies Award, the most recent user survey showed a satisfaction rate of 61 percent for physician users, 79 percent for allied health users, and 81 percent for nursing users, resulting in an overall satisfaction rate of 72 percent. The features physicians liked best included easy retrieval of clinical data, such as laboratory test results, access to the electronic patient record from any location, ease of entry of common orders, and useful printouts like Quick Scan.

TECHNOLOGY

In the acute care setting, Queen's ACIS included hardware architecture running key applications as follows:

- The mainframe incorporated an IBM ES9000 Model 622 with Eclipsys 7000, and permanent patient record database running in a dedicated logical partition with Pharmakon pharmacy management system and SMS Invision ADT system (with its proprietary database) running in separate partitions;
- IBM RS6000 running CoPath pathology system;
- IBM RS6000 running the Eclipsys enterprise data warehouse (EDW) on the Oracle platform;
- DEC VAX running IDX Radiology information system and Antrim Lab; and
- IBM RS6000 running the Datagate and Open Hub integration systems.

Operational data for acute care was stored centrally on RAID 5 and direct access storage devices (DASD) on the mainframe for availability 24 hours a day, seven days a week.

For ambulatory care, Queen's built the MedicaLogic EMR into a new architecture with Citrix WinFrame, a special configuration that allowed the end user to operate with a thin Citrix client on nonstandard PCs.

Security and data integrity were essential to Queen's ACIS. The mainframe and major servers were housed in a secure and environmentally controlled computer facility. Data backup occurred regularly on media stored off site. Key servers had sophisticated error detection, mirror functions, instant hot swap features, and redundancy upgrades to provide around the clock availability.

Two redundant LANs and smart hubs served each clinical area to ensure at least half the workstations in each unit would function during a LAN failure. Workstations were located in high visibility areas and locked to desks. Virus protection software ran automatically.

Finally, the ability to perform detailed electronic audits of access to the electronic record greatly strengthened Queen's confidentiality process. Audits were performed more frequently and efficiently. Publicizing results within the organization heightened awareness of the need for absolute confidentiality of patient records.

VALUE

Queen's defined ROI in its new ACIS as added value, where value meant measurable improvements in quality accompanied by significant cost savings. Central to the Queen's EHR initiative was the belief the greatest benefit would be achieved only if a critical mass of physicians used CLiQ in patient care. By the end of the first three years, some 60 to 63 percent of physicians were entering orders directly into the EHR.

Quality improvements included reductions in both the manual processing of orders and in medication turnaround time from drug order to administration. For STAT medication orders, the average turnaround time dropped by 20 percent. In the surgical intensive care unit (ICU), the mean time from order conception to order entry decreased by 57 percent. Improvements in compliance with Joint Commission on Accreditation of Healthcare Organizations (JCAHO) standards for restraint orders and for new allergy and advance directive guidelines were direct results of data collected and communicated by CLiQ. Further, since full activation of CLiQ in November 1995, medication errors decreased yearly.

Queen's original cost savings goal was for CLiQ and EDW to pay for themselves within five years and generate $10 million per year in cost savings after the fifth year. Queen's organized a CLiQ benefits study to measure progress. The model and results were verified by an independent consultant.

The study found Queen's case mix index increased significantly from 1994 through 1997, indicating care for progressively sicker patients during the study years. Savings occurred in laboratory, pharmacy, imaging, and other categories (mainly personnel). Cost savings were greater for variable costs than for fixed costs. The study estimated cost savings for the first three years after CLiQ and EDW implementation at approximately $66 million.

By focusing on clinical performance improvement rather than simply on computer technology, Queen's was able to integrate the EHR into the organization's clinical culture. The effort required listening, planning, collaboration, teamwork, and a willingness to embrace new ideas and technology. Results achieved included significant cost savings, better decision-making, and most importantly, improvements in patient care.

2000 DAVIES ORGANIZATIONAL AWARD WINNER
HARVARD VANGUARD MEDICAL ASSOCIATES
in partnership with Harvard Pilgrim Health Care

ABOUT THE ORGANIZATION

Harvard Vanguard Medical Associates (Harvard Vanguard) is a clinician-led, multi-specialty group practice with 14 locations in the greater Boston area serving 300,000 patients. It was formed in 1997 from the staff-model, health center-based operation of Harvard Community Health Plan. At the time it won the Davies Award, Harvard Vanguard had 600 physicians, 1,200 providers, and 2,100 support staff.

The majority of Harvard Vanguard's patients are members of the health maintenance organization that partnered in the Davies Award-winning computerized patient record (EHR) effort, Harvard Pilgrim Health Care, which serves 1.2 million members in the New England region. Key ties at the board of trustee level exist between the two organizations, and the EHR project represented a collaborative partnership over a long period of time.

Harvard Vanguard is a key fixture in the communities it serves, with long-standing patient relationships and loyalty maintained over a 30-year period. Its predecessor organization was one of the earliest users of a computer-based patient record in the country, serving as the initial installation site of an ambulatory patient record system (COSTAR) developed at Massachusetts General Hospital during the 1960s. By the late 1970s, the automated medical record system (AMRS) was a proprietary derivative of COSTAR and functioned as the glue during the early 1980s that enabled the predecessor organization to support care to the same patient at multiple locations.

MANAGEMENT

Limitations to the AMRS, whose underlying technology was predicated on 1960s and 1970s approaches to development, became apparent during the 1980s as clinicians sought more flexibility to incorporate and exploit guidelines and reminders. An initiative to develop a replacement application internally followed, but was halted after three years due to its unlikely successful completion.

An initiative to evaluate commercially available EHR systems followed, culminating in the selection of EpicCare from Epic Systems Inc., Madison, Wisconsin, in 1994. By 1996, implementation was completed at the initial 1996 pilot sites. Implementation at Harvard Vanguard's additional multi-specialty practice sites began in 1997. Installation at the final site and more than 100 affiliate locations, including hospitals and physicians offices throughout the Northeast region, was completed at the end of March 2000. The system was used by all Harvard Vanguard caregivers and clinical support staff.

System requirements documentation was voluminous, benefiting from 25 years of experience with computerized records and the abortive efforts at in-house development of an EHR. Key business requirements for an EHR included conversion and mapping of 25 years of patient data into the new EHR intact, flexibility to establish variable work flow to meet operational needs of individual practice sites, and shifting from a terminal-based environment to a PC-based workstation, among others. Of the 20 potential vendors, only Epic Systems met or exceeded functionality thresholds.

The four goals for the EHR included:

- To improve patient care by informing clinicians when tests were ordered, but not conducted, reminding clinicians when follow-up tests or monitoring were due, and other such reminders;
- To ultimately reduce paperwork for clinicians and allowing them to integrate and streamline scheduling, patient records, and billing;
- To replace an increasingly unreliable automated medical record system; and
- To support the aspects of the practice that made Harvard Vanguard's practice distinctive.

Organization leaders also expected the new CIS to pay for itself through such paybacks as reduced maintenance cost on the AMRS. The critical component in the cost justification was the expectation the costs of purchased care would be reduced 1.5 percent over the depreciated life of the application.

The EHR implementation project team, including training experts, work flow, implementation and system configuration analysts, clinician consultants, and programmers, ranged from 20 full-time equivalents (FTEs) to 30 FTEs as the implementation progressed. Each site also had its own implementation team. Three clinician workgroups helped to adapt, augment, standardize, and modify the application to support Harvard Vanguard's practices.

The approach to training clinicians and support staff combined the use of computer-based training, classroom training, departmental education sessions, work flow walk-throughs, individual coaching, and five-week, onsite post-go-live support. The intent was to give the users as many opportunities as possible to touch the system prior to the go-live date in their respective site(s).

Harvard Vanguard assured security and confidentiality through confidentiality agreements with employees, reminder messages, assignment of security classes, unique log-on identifiers, audit trails, password verification, and other methods.

FUNCTIONALITY

Data accessible through EpicCare included diagnoses, procedures, evaluation and management codes, medical or surgical history, historical information from the AMRS system, orders, results, immunization data, free-text clinical notes, telephone encounter information, medication lists, problem lists, health maintenance qualifiers, demographic information, allergy information, annotated images for encounters, and other information.

Harvard Vanguard used the entire integrated suite of application products from EpicCare, resulting in a core practice management system. Clinicians were required to enter and code diagnosis information, orders, and procedures. The system supported multiple options for data entry by users, including customized templates and macros to build notes rapidly during the course of the patient encounter. Interfaces with other data systems automatically posted data into the EHR.

Decision support tools offered to clinicians were extensive, including such features as health maintenance alerts, best-practice alerts, algorithms for medication substitutions, SmartSets for routine and acute care that automated required documentation, prescription writing, laboratory review, encounter searches, real-time recording of telephone encounters, and home and hospital access.

The key thread of all tools was dynamic access against current information in the patient's chart, warnings and rationale to the clinician at the point of care, and the opportunity to provide clinical intervention, such as ordering the necessary testing or medication, with a few keystrokes.

The EHR system was available for access from all 14 Harvard Vanguard sites and by remote access via PC/workstation. At the time of the award application, 2,700 individuals on average were using the system concurrently at any given time.

The EHR enhanced user-generated communications, but also allowed for system-generated automatic communication to users in appropriate contexts.

User satisfaction was significantly positive, related to several factors including availability of data, ease of use, wide use of the system, and availability of new capabilities. Early user surveys indicated most providers were able to produce at least the same number of patient visits while using the EHR, and overall, patient visits increased by 5 percent while the EHR was in use. A survey at the halfway point in the implementation indicated 72 percent of physicians reported the number of patients seen with the EHR equaled the number seen with AMRS, and an additional 8 percent were seeing more patients per session with the new system.

TECHNOLOGY

Harvard Vanguard used the Epic suite of products, with comprehensive computer-based patient record EpicCare. The integrated set of products supported demographic information for approximately 300,000 members, and supported, on an annual basis, clinical documentation for nearly 1.4 million patient visits, scheduling of nearly 1.8 million appointments, 1.9 million laboratory orders and results transactions, 2.5 million prescriptions, registration and coverage records for 1.4 million, and accounts receivable management for 5.1 million transactions, among other items.

Implementation of EpicCare required a complete upgrade of the organization's WAN, the implementation of LANs in all delivery sites, and the deployment of desktop PCs to all users. Migration from the existing MUMPS-based record to the new EHR and the conversion of 25 years of data required extensive planning.

System requirements included specified scalability, availability and reliability, security management and privacy, discrete data/data model, and integration.

Epic applications used ANSI-M technology, which was also the database and file system technology used by Harvard Vanguard's legacy EMR, AMRS. The software ran on Windows 3.1 and a DEC Alpha-based server running a nonstandard version of NT.

The system used a single Compaq Alpha 8400 server running cache to support nearly 3,000 concurrent users and 25 years of patient and medical data. The production environment had two identical Compaq Alpha 8400s with eight CPUs running at 525 megahertz (MHz) each. Only one Compaq Alpha 8400 was active at any one time, but a hot standby machine was available if the active machine had a hardware problem. The PC workstations used by all of the practice sites ranged from a 100MHz Pentium to a 400MHz Pentium, using at least 64MB of memory.

Security design features, based on a multi-level structure, included system registration, password-protected user login, and protected sets of access parameters.

The EHR used HL7 for exchanging order, result, transcription, pharmacy, and other information with non-Epic systems. The system was available 24/7, with the exception of a five-minute window at 11:00 p.m. when the system created a quiet point to freeze the transactions for backup.

VALUE

The estimated costs of implementing the EHR were approximately $21.5 million, or 1.2 percent of total gross revenue between 1997 and 2000.

The effect of implementation and use of the EHR system was profound and positive for the organization, clinicians, patients, partners, affiliates, and costs.

Following implementation, clinicians were able to access and enter information for Harvard Vanguard's 300,000 patients in all 14 practice sites and affiliate locations. Early user surveys indicated significant satisfaction with the EHR; nearly 80 percent of users agreed the system enabled them to retrieve data simply, quicker, and accurately; and 77 percent agreed the system helped them to better coordinate their patients' care.

Use of the EHR contributed to the effective delivery of care in four key ways: ready availability and accessibility of patients' records supported the provision of high quality care; accessibility of patients' records at key affiliate locations facilitated effective care delivery; legibility and completeness of prescriptions improved; and notification of abnormal findings also improved.

The EHR provided the underpinning for clinical management of population-based interventions for Harvard Vanguard. Already recognized for achieving nationally high Health Plan Employer Plan Data and Information Set (HEDIS) scores, the organization expected to hold these gains, add new performance measures, and target further health status improvement initiatives.

Harvard Vanguard's leaders concluded as follows: "Harvard Vanguard is now well positioned to continue to expand the use of this comprehensive tool (EHR) much more in the areas of clinical practice guidelines and decision support, further improving practice operations and efficiency, and clinical data reporting in general. The potential gain from using this electronic tool to improve the quality of care, improve each patient's health status, and impact cost is enormous."

2000 DAVIES ORGANIZATIONAL AWARD WINNER
VETERANS AFFAIRS PUGET SOUND
HEALTH CARE SYSTEM

ABOUT THE ORGANIZATION

The Veterans Affairs (VA) Puget Sound Health Care System, which includes two large medical center campuses, outpatient clinics, nursing homes, mental health facilities, and rehabilitation units, provides healthcare services for approximately 40,000 veterans in Washington.

In a project that began in 1997, VA Puget Sound implemented a computerized patient record system (CPRS) developed by the Department of Veterans Affairs to support entry of notes and orders, rules-based order checking, and results reporting.

VA Puget Sound served as the critical site for testing this software in a complex setting prior to its implementation throughout all 168 VA medical centers, outpatient clinics, and domiciliaries. CPRS software is layered on top of a large collection of applications and M databases used throughout the VA system.

At the time VA Puget Sound won the Davies Award, 850 physicians, 668 nurses, and a large number of other health professionals were using the CPRS as the primary medical record in all VA Puget Sound facilities and units.

MANAGEMENT

VA Puget Sound commenced its effort to implement a computer-based medical record system in February 1997 in order to meet three objectives: to improve the accessibility and availability of medical information wherever care was delivered; to support integrated care delivery to veterans at two divisions 40 miles apart and in the eight VA facilities in the Northwest network; and to benefit from improvements in care quality demonstrated at pioneering computer-based record system sites. At the same time, the organization needed to improve efficiency of care so costs were not increased (and possibly decreased) while improving the quality of care.

VA Puget Sound leadership was fully committed to the CPRS project and was willing to devote the necessary resources. The organization began assembling an implementation team, in fact, even before applying to become a test site, and successfully competed to be the third and largest test site for the CPRS software.

On winning the bid, VA Puget Sound formed a CPRS Steering Committee, comprised of senior clinical and administrative leaders from every discipline in the medical center, and two special groups of users—Clinical Champions, 20 clinicians who would advocate for an automated record, and super users who would receive more training than other users in order to coach others.

The organization also created a new entity to support the project, Clinical Information Management, and allocated 10 FTEs, clinical application coordinators

(CACs), to support CPRS implementation. CACs had clinical backgrounds and were able to provide thorough and high-quality user support.

All activities were undertaken with the full participation of representatives from the collective bargaining unit at VA Puget Sound.

VA Puget Sound planned CPRS installation to achieve two goals: to test features in the appropriate setting so developers could identify and address problems, and needed enhancements; and to achieve the defined user support standards.

Implementation was planned to occur in six waves at geographically grouped locations. It began on September 5, 1997 and was completed on October 5, 1999, encompassing all ambulatory care areas, all wards (excepting the bone marrow transplant unit), offices, and ancillary areas.

The first implementation step involved installing more than 2,000 desktop Windows NT workstations in patient care areas, offices, clinic exam rooms, and other locations where an automated medical record was likely to be used.

From day one of the first wave, all practitioners at VA Puget Sound could use CPRS to review results and to enter notes and consultations. Many practitioners adopted this new technology immediately, and the number of notes entered each day began climbing in a nearly linear fashion. Practitioners could enter notes either directly into CPRS, through a third-party note or report generation software, or through dictation, with subsequent upload into CPRS.

Automated practitioner order entry into CPRS was introduced on clinical units and required from that point on.

CPRS training, which began during implementation in groups of 20 users, changed to small-group training sessions as more users were trained and the software evolved. User support was provided 24 hours a day, 7 days a week, through CAC staff carrying pagers to respond to CPRS help pages.

Security and confidentiality procedures included user agreements signed by each user, education about security and confidentiality practices, and log-on authentication. Access to CPRS was controlled using a four-level control system.

FUNCTIONALITY

CPRS system functionality was organized into nine tabs that corresponded with those in the paper chart: cover sheet, problem list, medications, orders, notes, consults, discharge summaries, labs, and reports. CPRS brought together data for review from the majority of departmental systems containing clinical data on patients receiving care at VA Puget Sound. Data from other VA medical centers in the Pacific Northwest could be viewed by authorized users by using CPRS across the WAN.

Images that could be viewed through CPRS included radiographic images, ECGs, and digital dermatology clinic photographs. Endoscopic, pathology, and scanned document images were to be made available in the future.

Clinicians could enter orders into CPRS through one of three mechanisms, each of which offered advantages in certain settings: an ordering dialog screen; orders prepared in advance as quick orders that could be selected with a single click of the mouse or edited; and order sets that linked quick orders in sequence to generate many orders quickly.

CPRS note entry capabilities included note titles with associated templates and using the ad hoc templating capability, which allowed users to add information into any current note template they created or into those created for them.

Practitioners directly entered all consults, which were received and processed electronically by the consult receiving service.

CPRS was available to authorized users at the two VA Puget Sound campuses from approximately 2,200 Windows NT workstations available in all clinical areas, most offices, and conference rooms. All physicians whose credentials permitted them to care for VA Puget Sound patients were eligible to use dial-up access.

CPRS decision support features included:
- Order sets and quick orders to guide practitioners toward appropriate orders;
- Order checks for drug-drug, drug-disease, drug-food, and other interactions to reduce adverse medication events;
- Reminders to prompt users to order needed preventive and chronic care according to VA algorithms;
- View alerts and notifications that brought messages to the attention of clinicians;
- Clinical event monitors that scanned electronic messages to detect and prevent medication errors and notify appropriate groups when patients were admitted or transferred;
- Note templates that guided practitioners to gather required information; and
- Implementing guidelines that provided reminders to prompt clinicians to follow preventive and chronic care guidelines.

Clinician users at VA Puget Sound embraced CPRS. By January 2000, more than 3,300 notes were being entered each weekday and the repository contained more than 1.6 million electronic documents. By that same month, roughly two-thirds of all orders entered in outpatient and inpatient units combined were entered directly by practitioners. By the time of its Davies Award application, more than 10,000 orders were being processed each weekday.

TECHNOLOGY

CPRS had two front ends: the List Manager roll-and-scroll version that could be used from a terminal or by using terminal-emulating software on a PC, and the GUI, which required a Windows 95, 98, or NT workstation.

CPRS could be considered a semi-thick client at the top of a three-layer large collection of integrated Veterans Health Information Systems & Technology (VISTA) applications and databases. The deepest level consisted of the M databases running on the VISTA servers. The second level was the remote procedure call (RPC) broker that ran on both the server side and the client side, allowing communication between servers and clients.

The CPRS client was an application written in Delphi (object Pascal programming language) that ran on workstations running Windows 95, 98, or NT. The hosts running the server side were clusters of Compaq Alpha machines.

Although CPRS was the main software, it was not the only package used with the computerized patient record at VA Puget Sound. Other VA-developed software, such as

Bar Code Medication Administration and VISTA Imaging, and commercial software, such as Pulmonary Laboratory Reporting and Clinical Notes Template, were also used.

Security and data integrity were assured through VISTA's VA FileMan, Kernel, TaskManager, and other components. Messages sent between the VISTA applications and CPRS used the HL7 protocol.

VALUE

Documentation of the success in achieving VA Puget Sound's main objectives when launching the CPRS project—to supply providers with the information needed at the time and location of care, to support integrated care delivery at diverse locations, and to improve the quality of care—was commencing at the time of the organization's Davies Award application. Informal evaluation of the CPRS installation indicated the following encouraging results.

Documentation (and presumably delivery) of preventive care, such as prostate cancer screening and education, and alcohol screening, increased steadily following implementation of the CPRS. Compliance with acute care guidelines also improved, achieved in part through significant focus on order sets and order screens. The positive change in ordering practices was being sustained over time. Nursing and pharmacy staff reported that orders written using CPRS were uniformly easier to interpret than paper orders.

The clinical event monitor proved to be a valuable tool for clinicians and quality management groups charged with improving medication safety. On a typical day, the event monitor received 4,758 messages, 4,663 of which pertained to medication orders.

Reviews of charts from discharged inpatients conducted each month by the nursing department noted substantial and sustained increase in the documentation of assessment and delivery of care in accordance with VA Puget Sound policies and those of external review organizations. For example, documentation of clinical justification and rationale for the use of restraint and/or seclusion improved. The timeliness of chart completion post patient discharge from the hospital also improved.

VA Puget Sound leaders concluded, "The hard work and institutional commitment necessary to bring the VA CPRS into use at VA Puget Sound was worth the effort, and we look forward to the continuing benefits of having an electronic medical record."

2001 DAVIES ORGANIZATIONAL AWARD WINNER
HERITAGE BEHAVIORAL HEALTH CENTER, INC.

ABOUT THE ORGANIZATION

Heritage Behavioral Health Center is a private, not-for-profit comprehensive mental health and substance abuse organization based in Decatur, Illinois. Tracing its origins to 1956, Heritage has a legacy of providing high-quality, low-cost services to residents of the greater Macon County, Illinois area, without regard to clients' ability to pay. Through a staff of approximately 200 case managers, clinicians, nurses, and residential care staff, Heritage specializes in serving clients with the most serious illnesses, who often live in extreme poverty.

Heritage offers a broad continuum of community-based services. Its mental health services are heavily oriented to case management and psychosocial rehabilitation and include a variety of short- and long-term residential services. Substance abuse services include detoxification, residential rehabilitation, intensive inpatient and outpatient, including methadone therapy, and specialized services for women, adolescents, and individuals involved with the criminal justice system. The organization also provides outreach, crisis intervention, and prevention services to area residents, working from sites such as schools and public housing facilities.

Heritage operates from four treatment sites and has staff assigned to several additional sites operated by other community service organizations. At the time it won the Davies Award, Heritage treated more than 5,000 people annually, with approximately 3,500 clients in active treatment at any given time.

MANAGEMENT

In the mid-1990s, Heritage faced the possibility its state contracts and Medicaid-reimbursable services would be subject to increased competition. Heritage's inefficient data collection methods and antiquated information systems rendered it poorly prepared for that competition.

As part of its strategic planning, Heritage committed to the development of an extensive, internal corporate information network, called the Heritage Network. At the heart of this effort was the creation of a computer-based patient record, an initiative code-named Project Jericho, which referred to the walls of information system inefficiency that would have to come down.

The development of the Heritage Network and the EHR began in 1995. Heritage's leaders established four strategic objectives for the EHR project:
- Strengthen the service delivery process by developing a computer-based patient record that enhanced client care and served as a tool for caregivers;
- Improve the efficiency of the information system by automating and streamlining data collection and initiating real-time data entry;

- Increase staff access to information; and
- Enhance efforts to improve performance by monitoring the quality of internal operations and meeting the increasing demands of external funding and regulatory bodies.

Working with an information systems consultant, an interdisciplinary computer services team evaluated EHR options and, in July 1995, recommended the acquisition of specific hardware and software, and the consultation and training needed to provide core functions of electronic mail group work, scheduling, clinical information management, and accounts receivable.

The team selected and successfully negotiated reduced pricing with hardware and software vendors. Estimated expenditures were approximately $500,000 with annual operating costs of approximately $125,000 for an initial internal Heritage Network of 80 workstations offering group work, personal productivity software, electronic scheduling, and the EHR.

Team Jericho developed the EHR and later provided oversight for all information management systems. This cross-functional team included case managers, clinicians, financial specialists, a secretary, team leaders, group leaders, the vice presidents, and the CEO.

Implementation was planned to occur in four distinct phases. The first phase created an effective electronic mail and group work system, the Heritage Network. The second phase centralized and automated appointment scheduling, combining six different appointment scheduling processes into a single electronic system. The third phase thoroughly reviewed and re-engineered the service delivery process and the functions that support it, including the creation of an integrated, paper-based clinical record. This phase overlapped with the final phase of developing the EHR, which involved extensive testing, among other initiatives.

Heritage developed and taught three levels of training, designed to take an individual through the rudiments of computer use. This training introduced staff to the Microsoft Word, Lotus Notes, and Lotus Organizer applications available on the network and culminated in the receipt of an internal e-mail address. By 1996, the achievement of top-level training status became a requirement for successful completion of probation and continued employment.

As the EHR project was rolled out, training became more extensive. Team Jericho developed five distinct curricula for the EHR project: the clinical help desk, client registration and scheduling, assessment, progress notation, and treatment planning.

As the EHR was phased-in, the paper system was kept in place until the electronic system was verified as working. At each stage of implementation, caregivers were given the opportunity to go back to the paper process if client care was being affected by the use of the EHR. At that point, staff could record information manually, provided they subsequently entered those data into the EHR. The staff quickly adapted to the EHR and within months, even those who had been dictating assessments and progress notes, began to enter data as data was collected.

FUNCTIONALITY

Prior to the Jericho Project, the poor quality of paper-based client records, which negatively impacted both client care and corporate finances, was of concern to Heritage leaders and staff.

Needed systems re-engineering began with thorough flow charting of existing service delivery and support processes. This effort identified numerous problems with the paper-based record, including differing record formats, multiple charts, and varied assessment and treatment forms and formats.

To address these problems, a task force developed a universal record format, a single assessment form, a single treatment plan format, and other documents that would be adapted to the Clinician's Desktop electronic EHR to support the processes for completing those forms. As elements of the EHR were rolled out, administrative functions were reorganized to reflect the increased ability to collect and process information in real time.

The EHR developed by Heritage was based on four software applications: Clinician's Desktop and HSIS (Echo Group), MS Word 97, and InfoScriber (Conundrum Inc.). These programs automated the functions of client registration, scheduling, assessment, treatment planning, service documentation, and medication management.

Client registration occurred when all prospective clients completed a common registration process at their initial contact. All information gathered during this first contact was entered in real time and then populated appropriate fields on subsequent screens.

The scheduling of a client appointment initiated the call for documentation and billing for service. The design of the system required the service be scheduled before it could be processed for billing. Scheduling information was generally entered in real time but could be entered after the appointment was made.

Client assessment was conducted by four different assessment teams. A single set of assessment screens covered all age groups, both substance and mental health assessments, and the requirements of funding bodies. Assessment information was entered in real time using a common set of screens for all prospective clients.

To address treatment planning, the Heritage EHR featured a single set of treatment planning screens regardless of the client's age or presenting problem, following the integrated treatment planning process developed in the re-engineering phase.

To ensure efficient and easy service documentation, screens with framed questions prompted staff to create documentation consistent with best clinical practices and regulatory requirements.

For medication management, Heritage incorporated InfoScriber, a Web-based technology, which let clinicians add, change, discontinue, or reorder multiple medications for a patient in one transaction. The software enabled automated electronic prescribing with formulary checking, posting of drug interactions, drug allergy screening, laboratory scheduling, and administrative tracking.

The decision support features of Heritage's EHR were extensive. Diagnostic/assessment support enabled clinicians to arrive at more accurate diagnoses by guiding them through the data collection process. Treatment planning support used a series of drop-down menus, sorted by presenting problem area, to guide caregivers in building a tailored treatment plan using language acceptable to the appropriate regulatory authorities. Service documentation support checked documentation before it passed to the billing function. Medication management support provided immediate formulary checking, identification of possible drug interactions, drug allergy screening, laboratory scheduling, and administrative tracking.

Administrative support provided by the EHR included caseload management tools and summaries, billing and statistical reporting, quality improvement/utilization review, and corporate compliance.

The EHR program was accessible to all caregivers on 140 workstations in the main headquarters building and from remote sites. Most caregivers had access to a workstation within their work area, if not in their office. Access was limited to need-to-know information through case-record and specific-field security levels within Clinician's Desktop.

User satisfaction was high. Case managers reported a 22 percent increase efficiency of the EHR assessment process over the paper-based process; clinical staff reported a 17 percent increase with the EHR process. Administrative and support staff were even stronger in their support, with the former rating the EHR assessment 60 percent more efficient and the latter rating it 40 percent more efficient.

TECHNOLOGY

The Echo Group products (Clinician's Desktop and HSIS) were housed on a server running Microsoft Windows NT 4.0 and Microsoft SQL Server 7. The servers' hardware consisted of 1GB RAM, 18GB hard disk mirrored storage, and a 24GB digital audio tape (DAT) backup.

Lotus Notes was housed on a server that runs Microsoft Windows NT 4.0, Lotus Domino Server 4.51, and Microsoft Proxy Server 2.0 firewall software. The servers' hardware consisted of 128MB RAM, 9GB hard disk storage, and an 8GB DAT tape backup.

Citrix Metaframe 1.8 was used to connect off-site locations to the Heritage Network. It is housed on a server running Microsoft Windows NT Terminal Server 4.0.

Heritage chose to lease equipment and replace it every two years. This gave the organization great flexibility to buy quality products, which had minimal system downtime due to hardware failures, but presented the challenge of replacing the hardware at a time convenient to end users.

VALUE

User surveys indicate Project Jericho achieved its strategic objectives centered around improved client care and increased efficiency, as outlined earlier.

The project also achieved business expectations. As a result of the implementation of the EHR, Heritage reduced transcription costs associated with the documentation of client encounters in the clinical record by 70 percent. Other major sources of savings for a three-year period included: $750,000 savings in cost of equipment, software, information systems staffing, consultation and training; nearly $150,000 in chart audit paybacks; $117,000 reduction in back office staffing for data entry, and other savings, resulting in a total three-year savings of nearly $500,000.

In its Davies Award application, Heritage's leaders concluded, "The project to develop a computer-based patient record has met or exceeded its goal of improving the quality of information management and, thereby, the competitive position of Heritage Behavioral Health. The EHR has already produced significant benefits to corporate operations. The team-based developmental process has produced a superior product that serves the delivery of client care. The EHR provides highly accessible information that is far more timely and accurate than the paper-based system. It also raises the quality of the care provided by Heritage through its clinical decision supports. Finally, it has also embedded into the corporate culture the value of teams in the design and implementation of mission-critical systems."

2001 DAVIES ORGANIZATIONAL AWARD WINNER
OHIO STATE UNIVERSITY HEALTH SYSTEM

ABOUT THE ORGANIZATION

Located in Columbus, Ohio, the Ohio State University Health System (OSUHS) is a comprehensive integrated healthcare delivery system, which includes the Ohio State University Hospitals, the Arthur G. James Cancer Hospital and Richard J. Solove Research Institute, numerous clinics, physicians' offices, the College of Medicine and Public Health, community-based Ohio State University Hospitals East, and Harding Behavioral Health Hospital.

In 2000, OSUHS supported approximately 850-staffed beds, more than 40,000 hospital admissions, 71,000 emergency department visits, nearly 700,000 physician office visits, and 12,000 ambulatory surgeries. OSUHS employed approximately 6,000 staff members, 700 attending and courtesy physicians, 557 residents in 54 training programs, and 800 medical students, and supported many additional training programs including nursing, dentistry, pharmacy, and the allied health professions.

MANAGEMENT

In the early 1990s, OSUHS leaders identified a computerized patient record as a key component of its overall strategic plan and the vehicle that would enable the organization to achieve six key goals: maximize the quality of care; maximize efficiency and communication; minimize costs incurred by the organization and patients; maximize access to information without limitation of time and space; maximize compliance with the requirements of various regulatory agencies; and maximize user satisfaction.

A needs assessment, which commenced in 1993, resulted in a recommendation to move forward with selection of a vendor-based solution for physician order communications, and a new results reporting system to replace the legacy results system. Siemens was selected to be the core vendor for the OSUHS EHR, and Agfa-Bayer was selected as the vendor for a PACS.

Governance evolved during the different phases of the project, but throughout each phase, key stakeholders, including physicians, clinical support staff, hospital administration, and information systems, were represented. At one point, a 10-member Physician Consulting Group met for 24 months to gain design and development consensus from their peers, while challenging information systems to build technical solutions that would support the goals of the EHR. Following implementation, a Computerized Clinical Information Committee, co-chaired by the health system medical director and the chief information officer, provided oversight for systems integration and improvement.

Implementation planning included operational planning, change control planning, infrastructure and hardware preparation planning, and end-user support planning.

The implementation process for all phases of the EHR was structured to account for the complexity of change. The needs assessment for a phase or enhancement of the EHR applied to anything from a user change request to a new departmental system interface. The information systems staff and operational liaisons determined the feasibility. The analysis of the request laid out the way it was currently done via paper or electronic process. The design showed the way it could be done to satisfy the request and was prototyped for validation by the requestor or committee. Detailed programming of the request by the information systems staff was the next phase and usually flushed out additional design and validation steps. Testing was quite structured and consisted of a technical information systems testing step, a user validation and testing step, and an integrated testing step for things like interactions with ancillary areas or the admitting system or document routing.

EHR phases came live, if possible, in a pilot environment. OSUHS looked for a pilot to be fully operational so the user area was not subject to a dual manual and electronic system. OSUHS leaders carefully chose pilot areas and like areas were implemented as soon as possible after the pilot.

The transition to new processes benefited both from inclusion of physicians in all EHR development and implementation stages and standardization of system functionality, which also incorporated the needs of unique users and environments.

OSUHS' Department of Educational Development and Resources provided training for use of all aspects of the EHR, offering multiple training opportunities, a variety of training tools, training as close to the live event as possible, and extended training for super users, among other techniques. A help desk team offered users phone support for all EHR-related applications. In addition, a full time, onsite support staff of "red coats" was available to support the clinical systems. OSUHS monitored implementation progress through user meetings and feedback from the "red coats" on the pulse of the clinical users.

OSUHS developed and implemented enterprise-wide data security and patient confidentiality policies and procedures with role-based access controls. Any OSUHS user with appropriate security access could retrieve all data stored in the lifetime clinical repository database, with the exception of data specifically tied to a behavioral health encounter.

FUNCTIONALITY

OSUHS's targeted vision for EHR functionality was expressed as follows: "Imagine: information at your fingertips; simultaneous access to information; guiding user compliance to policy, protocol, guidelines, and standards; cost, quality, and outcomes measures at a moment's notice; and real-time notification of patient allergies, drug interactions, and contraindications."

Processes targeted for improvement included reporting of clinical results (for example, labs, procedures, etc.), recording of clinical documentation (for example, admission, discharge, daily progress, medication/ intravenous (IV) charting, etc.), entry of physician patient care orders (for example, orders, requisitions, consults, etc.), and collection of registration and billing information. OSUHS staff defined goals associated with each aspect of process improvement and defined specific process improvement indicators.

Early in its development, the vision of the OSUHS EHR considered user work flow, data redundancy, and benefits. Planners determined individuals who provide the source of data would be responsible for entering those data. Therefore, physicians and caregivers—as defined by law and by OSUHS bylaws—who prescribed or documented care or treatment for patients were responsible for entering information into the EHR. Data could be entered by keyboard, phone, or voice.

OSUHS deployed a variety of clinical and business systems linked by a master patient index. Clinical systems included a clinical results system (Siemens), a physician order-entry system (Siemens), a bedside documentation system (Clintelligent Corporation), a discharge documentation and patient education system (Siemens), an online decision support system (Siemens), a PACS (Agfa-Bayer), and numerous ancillary systems.

The business systems were supported by a patient management and patient accounting system (Siemens), an outpatient registration and physician billing system (IDX Corporation), a patient scheduling system (IDX), an electronic signature application (Softmed), and numerous ancillary systems. Standardization was a core principal in the design of all clinical and business systems and processes.

The EHR data components included clinical data, business and financial data, and administrative data. Clinical EHR data included: clinical results (labs, procedures, etc.), clinical documentation (admission, discharge, daily progress, medication/IV charting, etc.), and physician/patient care orders (orders, requisitions, consults, etc.).

Decision support capabilities were extensive, encompassing both systems designed to facilitate best practices, and clinical alerts and reminders that warned clinicians about patient variables. Expert knowledge was available to clinical and support staff in the form of help screens and via the intranet and Internet. For example, help screens within order entry included chemotherapy dosing calculations, frequency occurrence times, and listings of order set members.

An internally developed information warehouse housed all historic inpatient/outpatient clinical and financial data. Its goal was to provide a central repository of consistent, reliable data to be used for reporting. Areas of emphasis included outcomes research, strategic planning, targeted marketing, and the revenue cycle.

A variety of communication technologies were used, including internal system notification, interfaced communication, automatic paging, automatic e-mail notification, automatic faxing, and printing.

TECHNOLOGY

The EHR system architecture had six core platforms that housed its major systems.

The Siemens system for order entry, patient management, results reporting and patient accounting was housed on an IBM Model 9672-R26 mainframe server with VSAM files and DB2 Relational Database. Its platform had redundant power, processors, network connections, controllers, internal disk connections, and other hardware to avoid system-wide failure.

The Siemens system for document imaging, security and password management, rules engine, file servers, and terminal servers was housed on a platform of multiple

NT-based servers. The platform for the IDX system for outpatient registration and physician billing was a VAX cluster running a MUMPS database. The Agfa-Bayer PACS system was housed on a Sun Enterprise 5500 server running an Oracle database. The internally developed information warehouse also ran on an Oracle database. SeeBeyond provided the interface engine.

The software application used to maintain the data dictionary was the common vocabulary engine, which ran on two platforms: an Alpha SQL Server, which was the user front-end where the data dictionary maintenance occurs; then the Alpha SQL Server pushed the data to the IBM mainframe where it was stored into a DB2 database to serve as the dictionary over the lifetime clinical record (LCR) repository. This structure allowed OSUHS to define and standardize terms on both a detailed technical level and a clinical level.

More than 80 production interfaces were in place to ensure data was shared across applications. As new systems were added and user interfaces improved, the desktop workspace environment was kept as consistent as possible by creating PC images. These images allowed a PC to look and act the same regardless of its location or user population.

System reliability had to meet stringent requirements; OSUHS set an internal standard of less than 0.1 percent downtime.

OSUHS designed the EHR to support large- and small-scale implementations, as well as emerging technologies and innovations. Several strategies, such as strict adherence to industry standards, were used to ensure scalability. Standards were also enforced by using vendor-based systems when available.

VALUE

Through the implementation of physician order entry, clinical results, clinical documentation, and registration/billing processes, OSUHS achieved the six original goals identified at the onset of the EHR project, and met and far surpassed both the business and corporate objectives.

OSUHS conducted a formal study to evaluate the EHR's benefits and the specific process indicators related to its goals, a high-level summary of which follows.

Related to the goal of maximizing efficiency and communication, OSUHS patients received more timely care; results from ancillary departments were more efficient and accurate; turn-around times between nursing units and ancillary departments decreased (for example, average turnaround times for IV medications decreased from 5.28 hours prior to physician order entry to 1.51 hours post point of entry (POE) implementation); and work flow was enhanced.

Related to the goal of maximizing quality of patient care, OSUHS' EHR provided comprehensive information access that improved patient care (for example, reduced turnaround times resulted in faster delivery of patient care); automatic defaults and displays improved efficiency; clinical decision support tools improved patient safety (for example, online medication charting eliminated manual transcription errors); and length of stay decreased in a majority of service areas.

In the area of maximizing compliance, OSUHS' EHR enhanced compliance with organizational policy (for example, by facilitating use of best-practice clinical practice guidelines); met state policy and requirements; and complied with JCAHO and Health Care Financing Administration (HCFA) requirements.

Related to the goal of minimizing costs incurred to both the organization and patients, OSUHS' EHR improved cash flow (for example, by allowing expedited payor payment from various payors through electronically posting payments to the patient accounting systems), and contributed to reduced overall costs (for example, by reducing adverse drug events and lengths of stay).

In the area of maximizing access to information, OSUHS' EHR enhanced caregiver access, which improved patient care processes; provided access to information for patient decision support and for research and medical education; and ensured access to electronic data for quality measurement and needed interventions.

Finally, related to the goal of maximizing user satisfaction, testimonials about the benefits of OSUHS' EHR indicate strong support and satisfaction. Physicians cited computer order entry was positively impacting the way they delivered patient care; both payors and patients cited the benefits of immediate retrieval of billing documentation.

2001 DAVIES ORGANIZATIONAL AWARD WINNER
UNIVERSITY OF ILLINOIS AT CHICAGO
MEDICAL CENTER

ABOUT THE ORGANIZATION

Founded in 1882, the University of Illinois at Chicago Medical Center (UICMC) is the largest state-funded hospital in Illinois and among the busiest teaching institutions in the nation. UICMC has a 450-bed hospital, an outpatient surgery center, an outpatient care center, and eight satellite facilities located within 20 miles of the primary campus. The medical center includes colleges of medicine, nursing, pharmacy, dentistry, and health and human development sciences, and a school of public health.

At the time it won the Davies Award in 2001, UICMC had more than 700 affiliated physicians, generated annual revenues of more than $300 million, and employed more than 2,600 people, including 1,200 nurses, to provide care during approximately 18,000 inpatient admissions and 400,000 outpatient visits on an annual basis.

UICMC was ranked in the top 4 percent of America's hospitals in 12 specialties. As a tertiary site for many complex medical procedures, it supports programs in neurosurgery, ophthalmology, oncology, cardiology, neonatology, and obstetrics.

MANAGEMENT

In the early 1990s, UICMC began work on a long-term strategic initiative aimed at more fully integrating services between a planned outpatient care center and the hospital. Planners understood the medical center would need to upgrade its information systems infrastructure and replace its legacy patient care system in order to be Y2K compliant, to improve the quality of care by providing caregiver access to longitudinal EHR and clinical information across settings, and increase the efficiency and effectiveness of those who delivered care, among other objectives.

The planning, selection, and acquisition of the computerized patient record, which became known as the Gemini Project, were driven by a central body of executive and clinical leaders called the Executive Management Systems Steering Committee. The Gemini Executive Implementation Committee (EIC) provided oversight for implementation planning and decision- making. UICMC ensured strong physician involvement and ownership of the design and planning process by designating a physician and information technology co-chair for each of the committees reporting to the EIC.

Early in the process, UICMC decided not to create its own clinical applications, but to look to the vendor community for an application that would allow enterprise-wide connectivity and clinical decision support capabilities. After extensive review of alternatives, in 1995 UICMC selected and sought board approval for Health Network Architecture (HNA) Millennium developed by Cerner Corporation. The system, with an estimated cost of $10.3 million for hardware and software, was expected to provide significant dollar benefits through supply cost reductions, reimbursement benefits, and revenue enhancements. The medical center added 11 people to the IT staff to implement and maintain the system.

The project's implementation mantra was "Rapid Deployment: Share the Wealth," which reflected the objective of quickly benefiting the widest possible cross-section of the medical center. The incremental introduction of functionality provided a steady stream of new value for users, which helped increase end-user support and enthusiasm. Deployment occurred first in the ambulatory clinics, with all clinics converted by June 1998.

On the inpatient side, a "big bang" approach was taken to deploy the greatest amount of functionality in the shortest amount of time. Conversion from the hospital's 15-year-old legacy system occurred in November 1999, with order and documentation functionality converted on all 18 nursing units during a one-week period. This conversion effectively merged the inpatient and outpatient continuum of care into one clinical data repository.

The overall approach to training was comprehensive, with a range of educational options available for end users. A computer-based training program, with individual courses that took between one and two hours for trainees to complete, became the mainstay of the Gemini training effort. Nurses and physicians were provided separate learning paths based on their educational training needs.

UICMC ensured data integrity and security, among other measures, by cleaning legacy data prior to loading data into Cerner's clinical data repository, appointing a data steward and a security administrator, and developing a gateway through which data from all departments were required to pass before being stored on the Gemini database.

FUNCTIONALITY

The primary objective of Gemini was to replace both the inpatient and outpatient paper medical record over a period of five years. Users were to include physicians, nurses, licensed physical and occupational therapists, non-licensed clinical support, students from the health sciences colleges, pharmacists, and clerical staff.

The transformation process began in early 1999, when WinStations were upgraded across the hospital to allow outpatient physicians access to the earliest longitudinal patient record. Physician and nursing staff initially began using Gemini for all inpatient order entry, medication administration records, and laboratory result retrieval.

In addition to providing instant access to a broad array of patient information, Gemini allowed caregivers to order a range of clinical and diagnostic tests electronically, and then view results as soon as they were available. Gemini's functionality also supported enterprise-wide improvements in clinical decision support through such components as one that alerted clinicians and pharmacists of potential adverse drug events and drug interactions and another that guided clinicians through the care and documentation process.

Functionality within Gemini was designed to enhance communication and teamwork between and among caregivers. Clinicians also could access the system to support patient education and communication.

Applications available from the desktop included, among others, radiology information system, CareNotes, chart tracking and deficiency, anatomic pathology, Gemini patient care system, inpatient pharmacy, laboratory blood bank, general laboratory, utilization management, medical records imaging, enterprise scheduling, and person management registration. Document imaging was an integral part of the EHR.

Gemini was accessible to all authorized and appropriate caregivers and staff throughout all UICMC facilities 24 hours a day, seven days a week. System use increased steadily following the initial go-live date in October 1997. A user satisfaction survey in 2000 indicated high user acceptance, with 70 percent of physicians categorized as enthusiastic adopters. By 2001, Gemini was experiencing average daily access to the system by 1,600 caregivers, and opening of more than 500,000 charts each month.

TECHNOLOGY

UICMC's technology staff built a client/server architecture from the ground up, using a Microsoft NT network, an NT operating system, and 2,800 WinStations, and more than 4,500 client PCs that were able to interface with non-UICMC PCs. The network included 185 Intel servers that delivered e-mail, application, database, printing, intranet, and security services.

System updates could be provided through the servers without having to reprogram each of the PCs, which were available in every outpatient exam room, at every nurse station, conference room, and physician office. Rather than store application software locally, UICMC applications were stored on 15 application servers and a predefined ghost image was distributed to WinStations.

The Gemini (Cerner) applications ran on two Compaq 8400 Alpha machines, using VMS version 7.1-2, UCX version 5.0-10, and Oracle 7.3.3.6 as the database. The Alpha's ran in RAID 1 mode with complete drive shadowing, maximizing system availability and complete system redundancy. Interfaces between UICMC applications were exclusively managed by an interface engine, running on an IBM RS6000 and UNIX operating system, and using HL7 standards.

Because access to databases outside Gemini were critically important in the clinical environment, a connection was assured from the WinStations to the Multum drug database and the CareNotes database, both of which resided on servers in the UICMC data center.

Every aspect of Gemini was designed, developed, and implemented to facilitate efficient, scalable support and take advantage of emerging technologies. The RAID 1 controller array supported the highest level of system availability possible. With complete system redundancy, UICMC was able to avoid downtime for even a major hardware failure.

UICMC addressed security through three strategies: user authentication, access control, and accountability. Application training was required prior to access being granted, and security awareness and confidentiality training were provided annually.

The user-authentication process was based on a third-party arbitration scheme and occurred when users logged into the system. Access control was based on who the user is, who the patient is, and the desired level of disclosure between the two. All relationships declared by a user as he or she accesses a patient's chart were logged and tracked as they were activated, inactivated, or modified, thereby ensuring accountability.

VALUE

The value of the Gemini Project was significant. Clinical practice clearly improved, as evidenced by the following examples.

The system saved the time of the medical center's nursing staff, freeing nurses to provide more direct patient care. Nurses spent less time on medication administration, allowing approximately $1.2 million of nurse time to be reallocated away from manual documentation tasks. Physicians spent 30 percent less time looking for charts. More than 5,000 annual radiologist hours were redirected to patient care, jointly attributable to film access as well as access to a complete medical record through Gemini. Physicians saved five hours per week in the review of resident orders. Physicians, nurses, utilization review, and discharge planning staff found Gemini allowed them to begin the care review process much sooner.

A complete medical record was instantly available when a patient presented for care, resulting in a 40 percent reduction in the number of patients seen without a medical record. Chart pulls decreased by more than 75 percent (from 2,000 to 500 per month) due to the availability of electronic outpatient records. At least 12 paper forms were eliminated as a result of the automation available with Gemini.

Communication throughout the medical center improved. Gemini's forwarding functionality allowed better communication between physicians and nurses for abnormal test results and patient phone messages.

Approximately $1.7 million in ambulatory clinic construction costs and $39,000 in annual maintenance costs were averted. UICMC was so confident in the Gemini system that UICMC built the outpatient care center without medical record storage space. This decision resulted in a one-time construction cost savings of $1.7 million, along with an annual maintenance costs avoidance of nearly $40,000.

In October 2000, UICMC and Cerner jointly conducted an assessment of the value produced to date by Gemini. The study revealed the total estimated financial value generated by Gemini from project onset to the beginning of 2001 was $3.6 million.

2002 DAVIES ORGANIZATIONAL AWARD WINNER
MAIMONIDES MEDICAL CENTER

ABOUT THE ORGANIZATION

Maimonides Medical Center, a non-profit tertiary care facility with 705 beds, is located in the densely populated and ethnically diverse borough of Brooklyn, New York. A major academic affiliate of the Mount Sinai School of Medicine, Maimonides is the nation's third-largest independent teaching hospital, training more than 400 medical and surgical residents annually.

At the time Maimonides won the Davies Award, the hospital had more than 4,600 nursing and other employees, and approximately 277 employed physicians who coordinated care with a network of nearly 1,000 community physicians throughout the borough. Discharges numbered approximately 37,000, emergency department visits were about 77,000, and ambulatory visits exceeded 250,000 on an annual basis. The Maimonides staff speaks more than 45 languages to support healthcare services for its diverse patient population.

Although Maimonides was renowned for the quality of its medical care and its history as the site of the nation's first human heart transplant, its information environment remained "in the dark ages" up through the mid-1990s. The organization's application environment was still dependent on 1960s legacy keypunch-based mainframes—well behind its competitors in this regard.

By the mid-1990s, a number of factors converged to create the need for a new business model, which required an EHR that would allow prompt access to accurate patient data, financial information, and knowledge-based decision support for improved patient care quality and outcomes. Key precipitating factors included pressures to respond to managed competition, New York's deregulated reimbursement system, and Maimonides' goal to expand rapidly into an integrated delivery system.

MANAGEMENT

In 1996, Maimonides' executive management made a commitment and allocated the resources—one-third of the medical center's capital budget, or nearly $42 million over seven years—for a strong information environment that would improve the quality of care, increase patient satisfaction, reduce costs, and position the hospital for future growth. The result was Maimonides Access Clinical System (MACS), a leading-edge EHR system that provided real-time access to comprehensive clinical information wherever and whenever needed.

Business and clinical information technology needs at Maimonides were intense and diverse. In addition to the general need for an organization-wide EHR system, three departments had specific electronic record and advance decision support needs: obstetrics and the emergency department, where high volume and patient acuity raised the risk profile, and ambulatory health, where the use of paper charts impeded the continuity of care.

No single supplier could meet the hospital's requirements or deliver a truly integrated EHR solution. Accordingly, Maimonides evolved to a modified best-of-breed EHR approach, using selected vendors that met physician and departmental needs while conforming to the medical center's interfacing, hardware, software, and operating system standards.

The result was the implementation of four distinct EHR systems from different vendors:

- Eclipsys E-7000 Inpatient EHR, deployed in December 1996
- NextGen Ambulatory Care EHR, deployed in August 2001
- E&C IPRob Perinatal EHR, deployed in November 2001
- A4 Health Systems Emergency Department EHR, deployed in March 2002

In addition to the EHR systems, feeder systems covered laboratory, blood bank, radiology, transcription, PACS, patient management and accounting, decision support, human resources and finance, voice recognition, and operating room functions.

The leadership team prioritized and tracked each IT capital decision, using metrics such as clinical success factors and investment payback to ensure an adequate business return. The team also identified project risk factors and implemented risk reduction strategies to address implementation credibility, resistance to work flow change, vendor relationship management, information technology infrastructure, and uncertainty related to CPOE success.

Committees were formed during the implementation-planning phase to collect data, modify work flows, and design and modify systems to meet the medical center's needs. The decision to backload or to convert patient data was dependent on the system to be implemented. A data management committee identified all meaningful data collected for quality improvement, external reporting, and internal needs.

Project governance involved creating an EHR executive committee, work teams, project sponsors, physician task forces, a nursing council, and user groups. In building the management information systems (MIS) staff, Maimonides hired physicians, nurses, pharmacists, and other medical professionals with recognized and respected clinical experience who had a history with and knowledge of the organization. Technical experience was considered a bonus.

Just-in-time, customized training was conducted by specialty or by department, using physician-approved curriculum. User-specific training was and continues to be available as needed. Users and IT held daily debriefing meetings to identify process or system issues and required enhancements, and to ensure users were acclimating to the EHR. The goal was 100 percent utilization of MACS by all healthcare providers. Leaders considered the approach to training to be the most important factor in MACS' overall implementation success. In transitioning to new processes, leaders recognized the need to balance process standardization with a degree of local flexibility.

Creation of the clinical command center was the second most important implementation success factor. Staffed 24/7, 365 days a year, the command center provides user support for the four EHR systems, and monitoring of system processing and interfaces; it is an integral part of ongoing education and quality improvement.

FUNCTIONALITY

Maimonides' approach to the ongoing management of paper recognized that going paperless would take several years. Teams implemented each EHR using a pilot or phased-in approach. Physicians and other caregivers made key contributions to MACS functionality, from defining its overall strategy to advising about very specific elements of work flow and screen design.

The MACS computerized record draws data from a variety of sources, and is used in every aspect of treatment and administration of patient care. An enterprise registration system provides the master patient index (MPI), registration, census management, ambulatory patient scheduling, medical record numbers, and patient billing. Data can be entered through standard desktop terminals, as well as a full spectrum of mobile data entry devices, including voice recognition for radiologists and residents. An integrated electronic document management and distribution system makes discharge summaries, operative notes, and other material available to caregivers. More than 2000 computers throughout the medical center ensure that trained and authorized users have easy access to MACS. System pathways and templates are tailored to meet each category of user needs and patient care situations.

All employed physicians, community physicians, and residents use MACS to enter orders online, to review drug interactions, ancillary results, and digital images, and to fully document and chart clinical information. Using embedded decision support capabilities, intelligent rules engines provide clinical staff with treatment recommendations, diagnostic guidelines, and suggested medication dosages. Ancillary departments access MACS to view the status of tests; nurses use the system to document clinical information, dispense medication, and select charge information. All users can retrieve appropriate clinical data and results, including users in remote hospital locations or community physician offices. A partnership with WebMD provides patient decision support and facilitates patient education. Aggregated data analysis and reporting applications are extensive and powerful.

TECHNOLOGY

The Inpatient EHR application runs on an OS390/2.5 IBM mainframe located in Leonia, New Jersey. The three other EHR systems are Intel-based and run on a Windows NT 4.0 or Windows 2000 operating system. The emergency department, ambulatory, and perinatal EHR systems are client/server by design, leveraging a multi-tiered architecture. Data modeling is consistent across the four EHR systems.

Maimonides uses many different technologies to achieve system integration and was an early adopter of interface standards. The medical center's design philosophy is grounded on the idea of transferability and clustered scalability, achieved through the choice of Microsoft clustering on a Microsoft SQL database and the Intel platform. Its open design strategy and client/server architecture positions Maimonides to adopt emerging technologies.

All EHR systems meet federal, state, Health Insurance Portability and Accountability Act of 1996 (HIPAA), and JCAHO security and confidentiality requirements. Access to all systems is role-based; users are granted access after signing appropriate waivers and notifications of security policies, and undergoing a comprehensive training session. System integrity is maintained in numerous ways, such as storing EHR data via MVS and mirroring to provide immediate verification and error checking. All data exchange interfaces have been developed using HL7 standards and protocols. The main hospital campus was wired for technology using fiber optic connectivity.

VALUE

Maimonides' leaders recognized MACS would be difficult to evaluate on a financial basis alone; improved patient outcomes and satisfaction, health service efficiency, and patient and information access benefits must be factored into the equation. To track tangible financial ROI, Maimonides used a vendor's strategic investment model. Between 1996 and 2002 cumulatively, the total EHR solution achieved a 9.4 percent ROI, a 3.84-year payback, and positive net cash flow by year four.

Other benefits included the following:
- A 68 percent decrease in medication processing time, a 55 percent decrease in medication discrepancies, and a 58 percent reduction in problem medication orders;
- A 20 percent overall decrease in duplicate ancillary orders, including a 48 percent reduction in duplicate laboratory/chemistry tests; and
- A 2.21-day (30.4 percent) reduction in average length of patient stay resulting from improved speed of diagnosis and treatment made possible by increased accessibility of clinical data.

These improvements enabled 32,168 additional inpatients to be served by the medical center, representing more than $50 million in increased revenue, one quarter of which was attributed to the EHR.

In summarizing the factors contributing to the successes achieved through MACS, Maimonides' leaders highlighted the programs and methodologies contributing to physician participation, buy in, and ownership. Other key factors included building a clinically-focused MIS staff, selecting appropriate vendor partners, conducting training to meet the needs of all user constituencies, and winning the support of key leaders and advocates. They concluded: "The result is an information system environment that has brought dramatic improvements in the delivery of patient care, while positioning Maimonides to continue to fulfill its mission as a world-class medical institution in the years ahead."

EVOLUTION OF THE HOSPITAL'S EHR TO-DATE AND LESSONS TO SHARE

Challenges
Maimonides has faced and continues to address numerous challenges related to the MACS since 2002.

In the area of support, maintenance, and technological issues, the effort needed to maintain service levels of its best-of-breed integrated technology approach continues to grow beyond the initial expectations of the hospital's leadership. The organization's ability to respond quickly to new user and clinical needs, resulting from the ever-increasing complexity of the technology environment, presents a continuing challenge. Likewise, the complexity of data from legacy systems and the need for its continued integration create additional difficulties.

To address these issues, a Standards Committee is called upon to reaffirm the limits and expectations of technology for existing processes and new project initiatives. This ensures a methodical, integrated approach to the adoption of systems and technology, and keeps IT from becoming overburdened.

Although the hospital is committed to the use of decision support at the point of care, its complexity and specificity (for example, non-critical alerts versus critical alerts; too many alerts or too few alerts) can bring about clinical issues. Clinical leaders must continuously balance evidence-based care with organizational consensus-based practice in decision support logic and EHR use. The use of technology to improve delivery-of-care processes and patient outcomes requires the regular review of current and emerging technology. User and program needs and expectations must be balanced and addressed appropriately.

The hospital addresses these clinical issues by embedding evidence-based care and consensus-based practice guidelines in MACS. The Medical Informatics Committee, which represents the expansion on the Physician and Nurse Task Forces, helps to ensure ongoing clinical standardization organization-wide.

In the area of regulatory compliance, Maimonides, like all healthcare organizations, must balance privacy and security concerns with the need to deliver information any time and anywhere. The hospital has increased the number of staff dedicated to meeting security and regulatory guidelines, including auditing and monitoring functions, and deployed appropriate technology, such as VPN and e-mail encryption. All of the hospital's best-of-breed EHR applications must have the same high level of compliance with regulatory and JCAHO requirements. This has involved a significant increase in testing and monitoring.

The increased reliance on IT also continues to be a challenge. IT must provide data for quality improvement and other metric-based initiatives, including operations and management needs. Self-service data-reporting tools, such as Crystal Reports and Business Objects, have been introduced to encourage user participation where possible.

To maintain economy of scale, but still meet increasing needs for interoperability and standardization, Maimonides limits version upgrades to supportable levels based on existing staff and maintains adherence to pre-defined system/technology maintenance schedules.

As in all healthcare organizations, financial resources are divided among competing hospital priorities. IT continues to receive senior management and board-level support, as reflected by the significant percentage of capital funds allocated to IT on an annual basis.

The EHR Today and Its Effect on Care

The EHR at Maimonides have continued to grow. Since its implementation in 2002, use of the ambulatory EHR has expanded to all adult and pediatric primary and specialty clinics, as well as to psychiatry services. The emergency department EHR now includes all aspects of patient management. Use of the obstetric decision support EHR has expanded to the obstetric clinics. Remote access to the records and PACS by physician and clinical staff has expanded as well.

Data from legacy systems, such as EKG, cardiology, cardiac catheterization, fetal monitoring, and obstetrics ultrasound data, continue to be integrated into the MACS EHR. A fully-integrated cancer center EHR, including a radiation oncology module, has been implemented, while a perioperative scheduling, clinical documentation, and anesthesia electronic record is being integrated with MACS.

Implementation of MACS at Maimonides has continued to improve not only the delivery of patient care, but also the quality and efficiency of the care provided. Since 2002, the continued use of MACS and the enhancements made to the system(s) have bolstered hospital efforts to provide safe and high-quality patient care. Initiatives and enhancements include: removal of unsafe abbreviations; integration of medication safety alerts in all EHRs; standardization of medication ordering pathways for pediatric and neonatal patients; establishment of evidence-based guidelines and protocols throughout the continuum of care; implementation of electronic medication reconciliation upon patient admission and discharge; implementation of electronic discharge prescriptions; implementation of screening and prevention mechanisms, including smoking cessation, pneumococcal and influenza vaccination, and pediatric immunization; and identification of the pregnancy/lactation status of female patients.

Maimonides has also deployed technology to enhance patient capacity management and patient throughput. Expanded use of the intranet/Internet supports the clinical, educational, and operational activities of staff, physicians, and consumers.

Lessons Learned

The process of documenting and showing the value of MACS has had, and continues to have, an impact on both the organization's efficiency and the delivery of patient care. It has facilitated senior management, board, and physician acceptance of funding allocations to information technology. In addition, the increased use of technology has provided Maimonides with new and valuable business initiatives, alliances, and partnerships.

The hospital's leaders offer the following tips to other organizations:

- Never try to implement two or more clinical systems at the same time, because doing so stretches resources too thin and creates confusion among users and staff.
- Don't go live during peak census.
- Do a pilot, where possible.
- Test the system and interfaces in a production environment before going live.
- Whenever possible, backload information from the paper chart before going live so physicians can spend their time caring for patients rather than keying in data that already exist.
- Ensure customized order sets and pathways have the consensus of the affected group of physicians, and do not represent simply individual preferences.
- Be sure alert levels are consistent.
- Monitor interfaces around the clock.
- Be prepared to conduct training and support around the clock.

- Know the tolerance of your organization when making the decision between a single vendor and a best-of-breed approach. Select appropriate technology that is a match for both the IT staff and the tolerance and expectations of physicians and other users.
- Do not underestimate the effort involved in process re-engineering, or its impact on the organization. Process re-engineering represents at least 50 percent of the overall system implementation effort.

Maimonides leaders indicate strong leadership is essential: "Identify at least one or two physician leaders who are respected both clinically and technically, and make sure that they are on board with the selected technology and recommended implementation process."

2002 DAVIES ORGANIZATIONAL AWARD WINNER
QUEENS HEALTH NETWORK

ABOUT THE ORGANIZATION

Located in ethnically diverse Queens, New York, one of the five boroughs of New York City, Queens Health Network (QHN) serves a population of 2 million residents through Elmhurst Hospital Center, Queens Hospital Center (QHC), 11 freestanding medical clinics, and six school-based health centers. Teaching hospitals affiliated with the Mount Sinai School of Medicine, Elmhurst and Queens, have a combined total of 771 inpatient beds and more than 42,000 annual admissions. Through nearly 750 physicians, and a total of 6,100 employees in 2002 when it won the Davies Award, QHN provided inpatient care, more than 1 million ambulatory care visits, and 45,000 home healthcare visits.

QHC is a member of the New York City Health and Hospitals Corporation, one of the largest municipal health systems in the country. Patients come to Elmhurst and Queens Hospitals with more advanced disease processes, complications, and comorbidities than the general population, often because they have been denied care in other facilities because of their inability to pay.

The EHR deployed in the QHN, launched at Elmhurst Hospital Center in 1996, supported the clinical activities of all 2,800 clinical staff members, with approximately 4,300 staff members and physicians accessing the system each day. In 2002, the EHR supported clinical care related to 3,000 ambulatory patient visits each day at the two hospitals and 19 off-site medical centers, including six school-based programs.

MANAGEMENT

Senior executives of QHN proposed implementation of an EHR to the medical staff leadership in June 1996 as an integral component of the network's strategic and business plans. The senior team viewed the EHR as essential to the development of an effective infrastructure from which to support the reorganization of care, the design and refinement of quality measures and reporting processes, and the practice of evidence-based medicine to improve management of chronic disease.

An EHR steering committee, comprised of senior clinical and administrative leaders, established clinical and operational priorities. The project was considered time critical, and thus, its various application modules were implemented in phases.

Initial phases, completed within six months of launch, included creation of a physical and data communication infrastructure, clinical work flow analysis, software customization, project team training, development of system documentation and training program and documentation, implementation of a provider training program, transition plan development and implementation, establishment of a help desk, and software implementation and support.

Implementation of the EMR was initiated throughout ambulatory care in January 1997—a mere six months from the date of its proposed use—and interfaces to the existing electronic registration, laboratory, and radiology systems were developed. Physicians immediately started using the system to retrieve clinical test results, place test orders, and document problems on the patient problem list. Enhanced documentation features were added to the system as they were developed.

By December 1997, physicians throughout ambulatory care were using the EHR to document diagnoses, conditions, procedures, drug allergies, and to write online prescriptions. This approach, which started in ambulatory care with physicians providing CPOE and documenting the problem list, was different from the usual approach of starting on the inpatient side with use of the EHR by nursing staff. By February 2001, ambulatory primary care services, which received priority focus, were practically paperless.

By 2002, the EHR network included 3,000 personal computers, located throughout the organization—in exam rooms, ancillary departments, and on inpatient units.

User training was provided for all caregivers and whenever a new feature or function was introduced. In 2001, QHN installed a computer-based training program. Training continued to be customized in groups or on a one-to-one basis as needed.

QHN assured system security and patient confidentiality through need-to-know access restrictions, password protections, and encryption.

FUNCTIONALITY

QHN developed EHR functionality to address four targeted dimensions of quality: patient safety, efficiency of care, effectiveness of care, and timeliness of patient information.

Physicians and other clinicians entered patient information on PCs. The software enabled field-level data control in both the order entry and result entry processes. Extensive system audit trails also helped to promote the use of the fewest number of data elements possible. Duplication of data entry was eliminated through system functionality that allowed patient information to be displayed in order entry screens, in result entry screens, and in multiple display functions.

In order to control the input of patient information, the system had specific fields in order and results screens. Multiple views of data enabled visual validation of the information across venues.

Decision support, work flow, and communications functionality included the following:
- Real-time alerts and information embedded into the order entry and order results processes;
- Applications customized by service, yet standardized across services;
- Electronic work queues to reduce reliance on paper and speed turnaround time;
- Data elements with specific storage locations and characteristics defined to facilitate the interdisciplinary sharing of information;
- Software standardization and reporting tools to improve communications across departments;

- Database applications designed to ensure compliance with regulatory standards and requirements; and
- Department-specific quality assurance tools.

The scope and breadth of the QHN longitudinal patient record was large. For each data element, QHN specified the functions to be performed, individuals permitted to perform order entry/data capture, and required controls. EHR PCs were available in every location where clinical documentation was performed. Specific EHR features facilitated access to clinical information. For example, the chart review function provided summary level, detailed, longitudinal, and encounter-specific data review for each patient. All patient data obtained from the two acute care hospitals and the 19 clinics in the network were displayed in the electronic record.

TECHNOLOGY

QHN's EHR uses the Ulticare/Patient 1 system then-owned by Per-Se Technologies, which was the New York City Health and Hospitals Corporation's software choice. This system offered the ability to manage clinical data in all care delivery settings while maintaining data integrity. Radiographic, MRI, and ultrasound images were available at any clinical desktop via a PACS system developed by Agfa.

The registration and visit scheduling systems (Siemens) fed admission, discharge, and transfer data to Ulticare/Patient 1, which then transmitted charge data to the billing systems for procedures performed in radiology, cardiology, and the laboratories. Laboratory tests are ordered online, and results are imported via bidirectional interfaces to instruments or reference laboratories. Ulticare/Patient 1 serves as the hub of the radiology system, transmitting orders to both the voice recognition system (Talk Technologies) and the Agfa PACS, and storing and transmitting reports received from the voice recognition systems to the PACS. With the exception of mammography (a capability that was added following the Davies Award application), QHN was filmless.

Clinicians log in from their PCs via an enterprise network using redundant LAN and WAN technologies with auto fail-over to the EHR. The primary method of clinical data entry was the use of the keyboard and mouse to interact with extensive menu-driven screens that are module, clinic, provider, and activity-specific. Clinicians access the EHR from 3,000 PCs connected via the enterprise network.

The EHR had a closed proprietary data structure that could not be accessed or manipulated by any user of the system. Ulticare/Patient 1 was scalable in the number of additional application processors that could be assigned to the system, as well as the total amount of allowed disk storage.

QHN used a LAN design model that emphasized backbone redundancy to ensure maximum availability. Data integrity was maintained through four redundant RAID 5 copies of the clinical data across the mirrored servers, thereby offering quadruple data redundancy across physically distinct hardware platforms. Data loss was non-existent during the first five years the EHR was used live at QHN—and has continued to this day, including during the massive power outages experienced in New York City in August 2003. No data loss has occurred.

QHN used Health and Hospitals Corporation's security practices, including server and network equipment security hardening, desktop standards, anti-virus protection, and intruder detection/secure access solution.

The EHR operated 24 hours a day, seven days a week with no required downtime for backups. Response time was normally less than two seconds.

VALUE

QHN's leadership team of physicians and administrators determined success of the EHR would be measured by creation or improvement of processes that affected patient care:

- Improved access to patient information;
- Complete, legible clinical documentation to support quality patient care; and
- Timely and accurate patient data provided at the point of service throughout QHN.

The EHR's design and development focused on re-engineering of processes to foster improvements and access to patient care.

The EHR enabled every clinician working in the network to collect and interpret patient information; and use of the EHR by all staff was required throughout all project phases, beginning in ambulatory care. The EHR served as a catalyst for the development of clinical practice standards across services and departments network-wide.

Online documentation by physicians and mid-level providers significantly improved quality and completeness of clinical documentation. Queens Hospital Center reported a 50 percent reduction in the number of pharmacist interventions in medication orders in ambulatory care because of the system alerts, and the improved legibility and completeness of the prescriptions. By 1999 at Elmhurst Hospital, 100 percent of certain performance indicators, such as patient problem lists, Pap smears, and others, were complete. In a survey of primary care physicians conducted in February 2002, physicians reported the EHR saved them time conducting various activities, such as looking up laboratory results and writing prescriptions.

The EHR's integration of a digital radiography and a PACS dramatically reduced the percentage of studies never read as well as the time required to issue radiologists' reports. The results of 100 percent image availability to clinicians included faster interpretations, less repeat x-ray exposure to patients because of misplaced films and duplicate procedures, and faster patient discharges.

Patient care improved as access to information improved. For example, the point-of-care availability of real-time patient information reduced the number of hospital admissions because of warfarin toxicity. Providers in the anticoagulation clinic had easy and immediate access to drug dosage and interaction information.

The QHN EHR positioned the organization to provide patient care that was safe, effective, timely, and efficient. Because of the strong patient information infrastructure, QHN could re-engineer care processes, coordinate patient care across the continuum of time and location, sustain multi-disciplinary team functioning, and facilitate performance and outcomes measurement necessary to improve healthcare quality.

CURRENT STATUS AND LESSONS TO SHARE

In 2006 Queens Health Network, as a public health system, continues to face the resource challenges inherent in providing care to an ever-increasing population of uninsured or underinsured patients. QHN's EHR is helping the system to successfully address the challenges of maintaining and expanding capacity. Through the years and aided by EHR capabilities, QHN has expanded from a system with two hospitals and three or four off-site facilities to one that today includes two hospitals and 21 off-site facilities, including six school-based health programs.

The EHR at QHN is "everywhere," used by physicians, nurses, social workers, pharmacists, laboratory and radiology technicians, and other clinical and non-clinical staff. Progress notes, histories and physicals, discharge summaries, and other documentation are accomplished by clinicians online. On a continuous basis, the limited few remaining paper-based functions are replaced by online functions.

Early "acceptance" of the EHR has been replaced by an "appetite" for the technology. The EHR's ability to make information readily available and accessible has embedded its value organization-wide. Clinicians and other staff want to be able to accomplish more and more functions and access more and more information online.

Initial EHR implementation goals focused on process improvements to enhance care efficiency and effectiveness. Building on the accomplishment of these goals, the EHR can now focus on improving patient outcomes through such initiatives as population-based disease management. For example, QHN provides coordinated care for the more than 5,300 patients with diabetes through tracking and anticipating individual patient needs and providing a planned, systematic approach to care of this chronic condition.

The lessons learned during development and implementation of the EHR at Queens Health Network remain the lessons it wishes to share with other organizations today. These are:

- Listen! Listen to physicians to learn what they need to take care of patients. Listen to explanations of patient flow and paper flow to understand how to develop EHR tools to expedite these processes. Listen to users and creators of clinical information to understand what is essential and what wastes time.
- Physician order entry is a realizable goal if a partnership is created between the medical staff and the project team. A return on the investment of learning a new system must be realized as quickly as possible in the demonstrated value of electronic patient information (timeliness, availability, legibility).
- While pilots are important for gaining trust and testing functionality, successful implementation of a comprehensive, interdisciplinary patient record requires a "big bang" implementation strategy. The department or service will suffer the same period of upheaval regardless of whether the new application is rolled out to 20 or 200 or 2,000 users. Furthermore, integrated functionality must be simultaneously implemented across disciplines to provide its full capabilities and benefits to users.
- The process of automating the clinical patient record is less about technology and more about change management. People generally have a fear of the unknown, and often prefer "the devil they know over the devil they don't." Users learn at different rates: super users aren't always super, even if they've attended multiple classes. They

also have varying degrees of tolerance for change. Some who are initially EHR enemies eventually come around.

- Use of the EHR moves the organization into the information age. Ironically, because of the priority given to physicians in EHR development, support and implementation, the medical staff is often more expert than the support staff at the language, complexities, and capabilities of the system. The organization insisted the clinicians work toward a paperless environment, while many of the mid-level managers continued to resist the role of super user essential to provide the first line of support for clinicians.

- The importance of physician leadership to the successful implementation of the EHR can't be overstated. Lack of enthusiasm for the project from the chief of service will guarantee limited satisfaction with and use of the EHR within a service. Differences are apparent across campuses and within services, where the application and the technology are exactly the same.

- System integration is the key to providing clinical information in the easiest, most expedient format possible. Foreign system interfaces require maintenance, troubleshooting and inevitably cause data integrity and reliability issues for clinicians.

- The development of clinical practice standards requires hard work and compromise, and they must be agreed to before system implementation. The EHR can't be programmed to follow certain rules, providing decision support in the process, unless consensus is reached by the medical staff.

- Keeping it simple and quick, especially for physician order entry functions, is another key to success. The project team must remember there are multiple customers for each application under development. It is important for system efficiency not to allow extraneous questions, inconsistent displays, and flashing reminders to clutter screens.

Queens Health Network achieved a rapid transformation from a paper-based organization to an EHR-based system, which occurred in ambulatory care over a brief six-month period and organization-wide shortly thereafter, in the years before widespread support for EHRs emerged from Congress, patient safety organizations, and other organizations. QHN expects to continue its leadership position in using the EHR to overcoming obstacles to integrated, seamless care across the entire spectrum of healthcare services.

2003 DAVIES ORGANIZATIONAL AWARD WINNER
CINCINNATI CHILDREN'S HOSPITAL
MEDICAL CENTER

ABOUT THE ORGANIZATION

Cincinnati Children's Hospital Medical Center (CCHMC) is a 324-bed tertiary care hospital serving a primary area with more than 550,000 children in Southern Ohio, Northern Kentucky, Eastern Indiana, and Western West Virginia, and secondary referrals from 42 states and 31 countries. Children receive care in CCHMC's multiple centers of excellence, including the solid organ transplant center, the heart center, the blood and marrow transplant center, the regional center for newborn intensive care, the aerodigestive center, and many others. In addition to its main campus in Cincinnati, Ohio, CCHMC has 15 off-site clinics.

In 2002, CCHMC admitted approximately 20,000 inpatients, and provided care during 87,000 emergency department visits, 577,000 outpatient visits, and 12,000 home care visits. Staffing included more than 1,000 affiliated physicians, 1,700 nurses, and thousands of allied health professionals. CCHMC trains undergraduate medical students, residents, fellows, nurses, and allied health professionals.

The Children's Hospital Research Foundation, founded in 1931, is a nationally recognized pediatric research institution, whose scientists have been responsible for such breakthrough discoveries as the oral polio vaccine and the first practical heart-lung machine that made open-heart surgery possible.

MANAGEMENT

In 2000, using Six Sigma's Define, Measure, Analyze, Improve, and Control (DMAIC) process improvement approach, CCHMC began the journey to integrate informatics systems technology directly into the work flow and clinical decision-making processes of physicians and nurses.

Within an 18-month period, CCHMC planned, built, and implemented a leading-edge electronic platform that included browser technology-based systems, computerized clinical order entry (COE), clinical documentation, electronic medication and intravenous charting, rules engine, and lifetime electronic clinical records. The industry standard for implementing such a system was roughly three years.

Named Integrating Clinical Informatics System (ICIS), the initiative had nine strategic objectives: optimizing patient safety; optimizing consistency in care; improving clinician and patient care efficiency; maximizing regulatory compliance; enhancing provider, patient, and family satisfaction; providing cost-effective care; improving the education of staff and trainees; enhancing research productivity; and strengthening performance improvement activities.

To meet these objectives, CCHMC's leaders recognized the need for COE and an informatics platform that fully integrated all clinical application, including the enterprise-wide PACS implemented in March 2000. Assignment of physicians as COE project director and as the medical director of information services (and PACS team leader) was the catalyst that ensured physician partnership and ownership.

The ICIS Leadership Team selected the INVISION system from Siemens Medical Solutions Health Services Corporation as the electronic platform for ICIS. Capital expenditures for server and software, implementation of a wireless infrastructure, fixed and wireless devices, and other associated costs, were approximately $5.3 million over a three-year period (2000 to 2002).

CCHMC took four steps to ensure the project's success: multidisciplinary ICIS users were invited to join one of two ICIS design teams; the hospital hired a consulting firm to provide project management and implementation services; a significant public relations campaign began 18 months prior to the first unit implementation; and the pilot units for implementing ICIS were carefully selected.

The implementation of ICIS required a multifaceted approach including work flow analysis, improvements in underlying processes, and a sound, user-friendly design approach. The ICIS leadership team was challenged with providing an optimal solution to meet the unique care needs of children. Detailed analysis of clinician work flow, with its associated process variations and inefficiencies in care delivery, identified the need for ICIS to provide a level of complexity that was not available in the proprietary software.

To meet the project's needs, CCHMC created numerous teams whose primary focus was to provide clinical input necessary to optimize the design of ICIS while ensuring the integration of ICIS into the clinical work flow. For example, Patient Care and Access Process Initiatives (PCAPI) teams worked with physicians, nurses, and ICIS project leaders to outline principles of change with the goal of standardizing process, improving patient flow, maximizing revenue capture, and ultimately improving patient and family satisfaction. Teams identified and championed the significant process re-engineering needed to make ICIS a success.

Several weeks of live implementation planning occurred before the introduction of ICIS in any patient care area. One implementation strategy involved ICIS usability testing by clinician advocates in an area prior to ICIS implementation in that area.

The implementation timeline was a rapid one—18 months. Organization-wide implementation of the Web-based portal occurred in August 2000; COE, clinical documentation, and Med/IV charting analysis and system design began in October 2000.

An ICIS education team implemented the public relations campaign, and ensured role-based and just-in-time training. "Blue coats" provided first-level support to clinicians, communicated ongoing functionality updates, and provided real-time focused training when and where necessary.

ICIS implementation was planned in a phased approach so the impacts on operations were well controlled and disruptions were minimized. Processes most significantly affected were those related to patient flow through the hospital. New processes for learning where to find the electronic data and how to read the new printed forms needed to be developed for both the ICIS and non-ICIS units to which the patient may be transferring to or from.

As a pediatric organization, every aspect of the implementation had to be analyzed in great detail to ensure system compatibility with children and their families. For example, portable devices had the potential to intimidate or scare small children. Loose electrical cords and non-stable carts could be dangerous to these patients.

FUNCTIONALITY

Functionality included in ICIS was designed to meet strategic objectives: safety, consistency, efficiency, compliance, user/patient/family satisfaction, and care based on research and performance improvement activities.

The COE application included all inpatient care orders, approved procedure, and diagnosis-based pediatric-specific order sets. With patient safety as the main driving force, standard decision support tools were employed, such as drug allergy, duplicate orders, therapeutic drug duplicate, and drug/drug interaction checking.

Additional pediatric-specific decision support tools were designed and implemented in various ICIS pathways. For example, due to the lack of available commercial dose reference data for children, and particularly for neonates, dose-range checking capabilities were critical. These were provided by a dose range checker, an application based on years of research at CCHMC.

The clinical documentation application included vital signs, heights, weights, allergies, physical and admission history, intake and output records, IV and central venous catheter assessments, and pain assessments. Nurse-to-nurse communication orders allowed nurses to select orders that were based on the developmental age of the patient (i.e., infant, toddler, school-age, adolescent, and adult). Admission history and pain assessment tools allowed clinicians to tailor documentation to the developmental age of the patient.

The integration of COE and clinical documentation resulted in the generation of the Med/IV charting platform, (the electronic medication administration record), directly linking the ordering, dispensing, and administration processing in the medication-management cycle.

Since ICIS was a Web-based system, information was available from any device within the organization, whether in the outpatient clinics, inpatient units, or one of the 15 satellite clinics. CCHMC encouraged clinicians to place orders from anywhere within the organization when patient conditions changed in order to minimize the need for verbal orders, and thereby reduce the potential for medication errors. A combination of fixed and mobile devices was deployed to meet user needs.

To provide decision support and enhance clinical practice standardization, ICIS contained 181 orders sets, 27 of which were best-practice guidelines, and 48 convenience sets. Other decision support tools included Internet-based and intranet-based resources, system help, and information screens.

ICIS made a wealth of information available for performance improvement activities and data sharing with other organizations. For example, ICIS aggregated data analysis and reporting functions included such capabilities as a disease-specific patient registry database, which was used in research and process improvement.

TECHNOLOGY

The ICIS client server production environment was built on two servers, running on two clustered servers. Each server was an HP LT6000r with six CPU (700MHz each), 8GB RAM. The operating system for each server was Microsoft Windows 2000 Advanced Server.

To minimize impact on the production system, a test and development environment was built on separate servers. The mainframe was an IBM model RA6, 88 MIPS size using OS390 R2.10, which stored approximately 1 tera-byte of data and processes, an estimated 500,000 transactions per day. It provided connectivity to 4,500 devices on main campus and off-site locations and supported the Siemens-based applications.

The ICIS Web servers provided Web-based services for the workstations using vendor's proprietary code. The Integration Engine - OPENLink™ ran as a client/server solution using an Intel-based PC server and required Microsoft Windows 2000 as the primary operating system. OPENLink™ used completely mirrored (identical) servers.

CCHMC's physical server infrastructure was comprised of HP/Compaq rack-mounted server hardware. At the time of the Davies Award application, there were 170-plus Windows 2000/NT servers and 50-plus Novell 4.11/5.1/6 servers. Windows 2000 was the primary platform for application servers. Critical applications/services were placed on clustered hardware to provide high availability. The ICIS applications were accessed via thin-client MS Windows-based desktops and laptops.

ICIS applications were continually undergoing upgrades and enhancements through the application of vendor updates and customization, as the business needs demanded. Vendor updates were carefully evaluated and tested prior to implementation to assure they provided value-added features.

VALUE

CCHMC tracked process improvement outcomes associated with the nine strategic objectives of ICIS implementation cited earlier. Significant positive outcomes occurred in each domain.

For example, in order to optimize patient safety, teams defined complete, unambiguous, and legible orders as one process improvement outcome. As a result of the ICIS implementation, clinicians generated complete, unambiguous, legible orders that included clinician contact name and pager number on all orders. Other gains included the decrease in number of phone calls to clinicians and the dramatically decreased medication turnaround time. Turnaround time improvements ranged from an 18 to 85 percent decrease in time, depending on the medication cycle stage.

Or, for example, in the area of optimizing consistency of care, the process improvement outcome use of order sets and clinical practice guidelines showed a 20 percent improvement in diagnosis of bronchiolitis—from 50 percent use pre-ICIS implementation to 70 percent use post-implementation.

CCHMC leaders cited ICIS' success as "likely attributable to a principle strategy of putting ownership of the system in the hands of the clinicians." Physicians led the project effort; physicians, nurses and other clinicians drove the design processes; and the organizational culture empowered all clinicians to embrace the system based on its merit.

CCHMC leaders concluded, "ICIS was instrumental in helping CCHMC realize its vision of dramatically improving patient care, greatly increasing the impact of research, and implementing new models of education for pediatric professionals, patients, families, and the public."

2004 DAVIES ORGANIZATIONAL AWARD WINNER
EVANSTON NORTHWESTERN HEALTHCARE

ABOUT THE ORGANIZATION

Located in Chicago's Northern suburbs, Evanston Northwestern Healthcare (ENH) is an academic health system that owns and operates three hospitals—Evanston Hospital, Glenbrook Hospital, and Highland Park Hospital—with a combined total of nearly 800 beds.

ENH also employs approximately 500 physicians in a faculty group practice, 284 of whom are community-based, and has a professional staff of more than 1,600 physicians who admit patients to the three hospitals. ENH admits approximately 38,000 inpatients, and provides patient care during 91,000 emergency department visits and nearly 800,000 outpatient visits on an annual basis.

ENH is a teaching institution, affiliated with Evanston-based Northwestern University's Feinberg School of Medicine.

MANAGEMENT

Although ENH's willingness to adopt and embrace information technology began more than two decades ago, in 2001 ENH's leaders established as the organization's number one priority the implementation of a paperless, patient-centric EHR, with true CPOE that would cover the three hospitals and 68 office locations.

The vision for the new paperless system included the requirement every physician and every clinician would use the system in order to meet the project's four goals: improving patient safety by eliminating problems associated with illegible orders and medication errors; ensuring physicians, clinicians, and administrators had access to the right patient data at the right time; ensuring the accuracy of the information and coded data in the record; and simplifying processes and making them consistent across the organization.

Following review of potential software vendors, in June 2001 ENH selected Epic Systems as the vendor that came closest to delivering on the ENH vision. Epic had the needed software, but ENH would be the first customer to implement a suite of Epic applications in a paperless environment across an integrated delivery system. Supporting seven operational areas, software included registration, scheduling, physician billing, inpatient and outpatient clinical documentation and orders, ambulatory (off-site) clinical documentation and orders, pharmacy, and emergency department applications.

Capital and operational expenditures from year 2001 through 2004 were $35 million. Savings were projected to be $60 million over a five-year period, resulting from lower receivables and staffing efficiencies, greater coding accuracy, fewer medication errors, and centralized scheduling.

Implementation planning ran on two parallel tracks: The first focused on hardware selection and implementation, and the second track focused on redesigning work flows and then building and installing the software to support these new work flows.

In order to implement a consistent set of processes, ENH first had to develop a consistent set of processes. Over a three-month period, teams with leaders in each of seven operational areas analyzed and redesigned every work flow process in the three hospitals. They then worked with IS staff to build the documentation in the Epic system that would create a single patient record organization-wide. For the 68 practice sites, the ambulatory team developed a basic set of standardized work flows to serve as a model for all sites.

ENH believed rapid implementation of the EHR created the greatest potential to reduce the number of patient care errors and improve the quality of care. As such, the organization chose a no-pilot, all-at-once approach to provide an integrated system as quickly as possible and to reduce the risks inherent with dual systems.

ENH implemented the system in two major phases for the hospitals—first documentation systems, and second, order entry systems—and similarly, two phases for the physician offices—first administrative functions and then clinical systems. ENH created a command center for each go-live phase in each hospital. Staff received extensive practice session opportunities in the three to four months before implementation in each ambulatory location. Go-live implementation in the hospitals started in March 2003 and was completed by April 2004; the first of 68 office locations went live in January 2003 with the final go-live date occurring in October 2004.

ENH made a massive investment in training, the goal of which was not just to teach the functionality of the software, but also to introduce all staff to the new work flows and radically new ways of performing their jobs. Everyone who touched the health record across the entire organization—more than 9,500 people—were trained an average of 16 hours each, and their competency verified. To admit to or treat patients in ENH hospitals, physicians were required to complete 16 to 24 hours of training and pass the competency test.

The data capture tools were built for ENH so the individual providing care entered data into the system once at the point of care. To meet this end, standardized rows within the flow sheet, the primary data capture tool, enabled the data to be entered through any type of template and be reviewed in the format appropriate to that user.

FUNCTIONALITY

The Epic-based system integrated functions across the organization, including ambulatory registration (Prelude module), scheduling (Cadence module), physician billing (Resolute), inpatient clinical documentation and orders (EpicCare Inpatient), ambulatory clinical documentation and orders (EpicCare Ambulatory), pharmacy prescriptions and medication orders (EpicRx), and emergency department (EpidCare ED).

The system required physicians and other clinicians to place orders electronically at the point of care, and incorporated the patient's care plan into the record and alerted staff to potential medical issues. Physicians, nurses, and all caregivers documented all the care they provided directly into the EHR using wireless mobile devices.

All of the modules (applications) functioned in a highly integrated manner because they shared a common database. Each encounter (office visit, phone call, emergency department visit, outpatient visit, and inpatient stay) was tied to an individual patient, and data from any and all encounters was available to clinicians who are responsible for the patient's care. Problem lists, allergies, and medications were available at every encounter, giving clinicians the most current information. The EHR was available in the physician office, the exam rooms, at 6,000 devices throughout the three hospitals, and at remote locations, such as from a physician's home, through the Internet. Remote access was provided through Secure Sockets Layer (SSL) encryption and secure ID passwords. Remote access was encrypted as it passed through the Internet for security.

The EHR included all eight of the core functions the IOM specified should be included in any EHR system: health information and data, result management, order management, decision support, electronic communication and connectivity, patient support, administrative processes, and reporting. As a result of the rapid staged roll out of these eight core capabilities, and only 18 months after its initial implementation, ENH was fully using all of the core capabilities.

Decision support universal tools available at all inpatient, outpatient, and ambulatory settings included: more than 1,000 physician order sets that help physicians place orders efficiently and follow best practices; medication and allergy alerts for all medication orders, allergy verification alert prohibiting order entry if allergy not documented within the past year; recommended doses for weight-based medications and age-related alerts, and many others. Tools available at ambulatory settings included prompts for health maintenance measures to promote wellness, and custom designed flow sheets by specialty to collate pertinent data for monitoring trends over time.

Knowledge access, patient education and support for care decisions, aggregated data analysis and reporting, work flow and communication enhancement, and data sharing capabilities were extensive.

TECHNOLOGY

ENH's goal in architecting the EHR system was to create a resilient environment using the latest high availability technology. The system was to be used 24/7, 365 days a year, and unplanned downtime was to be held to an absolute minimum. Using a system failover model, ENH incorporated redundant servers, storage area network equipment, and high availability software.

The back-end application and database system components included two IBM P690 frames with 24 CPU capabilities. Multiple fiber channel adapters accessed the storage area network on an IBM ESS 800 frame. Connections to the gigabit Ethernet (GbE) network were through multiple copper gigabit adapters. The high availability solution coupled the two servers using IBM's High Availability Cluster Multi-Processing (HACMP) software.

The then-current production system required 15 CPUs to accommodate the main production system, which uses 1600 Caché database licenses. Each 24 CPU frame had the capability to run 24 distinct environments if needed.

The applications and database were integrated and ran on the same back-end server. The client code was installed on a Citrix farm of 100 servers using Hewlett Packard blade technology. Users connected to the applications on 2,000 thin clients via a Web page called E-LINK, the gateway to the client software.

The wireless network provided point-of-care capability to physicians and nurses using the Epic-based system. The wireless network had more than 400 access points and was installed at all three hospitals. Coverage was at 100 percent in all of these clinical settings, which also accommodates the voice over IP (VoIP) phones the nurses used. Mobile carts, called "Jetsons" by nurses (after the 1960s cartoon), brought the chart to the bedside at point of care. The carts contained a terminal device connected wirelessly to the LAN.

VALUE

For ENH, the primary purpose of implementing the Epic-based EHR/CPOE system was to move the organization along the path of becoming the best-integrated healthcare delivery system serving Chicago's suburban North Shore. The success of the project in achieving that objective derived from four key factors: end-to-end process redesign before implementation, software functionality, end-to-end system integration, and 100 percent adoption across the organization.

Although implementation was just completing at the time of its Davies Award application, available statistical and anecdotal data indicated the new system was making progress toward achieving its original patient safety, access, accuracy, and process simplification and standardization goals.

In the area of patient safety, the new system eliminated entire categories of errors and near misses, including transcription errors, errors due to misunderstood abbreviations, and mix-ups due to look-alike drug names. The system also reduced delays and omissions in administration of medications, and assured continuous compliance with applicable National Patient Safety Goals as required by JCAHO.

Related to patient data accessibility and availability, point-of-care documentation was immediately integrated into the chart and available to all clinicians and members of the healthcare team. Physicians and other clinicians could access and update patient information wherever and whenever necessary. All health records were secure and password-protected, though instantly accessible to those who need to see them.

In the area of record accuracy and completeness in hospitals and medical offices, billing denials and returned mail both provided relevant indicators. With the new system, the overall billing denial rate dropped from 23 percent to 10 percent. The returned mail rate dropped from 5 percent to zero.

Simplified and consistent processes across the continuum of care were achieved by ENH through ensuring end users drove the improvement effort. The result was a robust set of more than 50 clinical pathways that logically extended seamlessly across the organization. ENH was unique in that its links created a continuum of care that began in the physician office, continued through hospital outpatient visits, the acute care stay, and back to the physician office for follow up. Clinicians could view a patient's progress and influence outcomes in real time.

At the time of its Davies Award application, ENH had begun to see improvements in several financial metrics. For example, the co-pay collection rate had increased from 21 percent to 50 percent. Physician office practices noted the system's potential to enhance revenue through better charge capture and greater billing accuracy. Staff-related cost reductions amounted to $7.8 million; other revenue and service-related cost reductions contributed to a total savings of more than $12 million in annualized costs.

As Arnold Wagner, Jr., MD, head of the Physician Advisory Group for the system concluded, "Evanston Northwestern Healthcare is showing how the innovative use of technology can deliver community-based medicine that leads to better patient outcomes. It puts the collective focus of our work right where it belongs—on the patient. And it makes Evanston Northwestern Healthcare a better place to practice medicine."

2005 DAVIES ORGANIZATIONAL AWARD WINNER
CITIZENS MEMORIAL HEALTHCARE

ABOUT THE ORGANIZATION

Citizens Memorial Healthcare (CMH) is an integrated rural healthcare delivery system serving a population of 80,000 in Southwest Missouri and headquartered in the town of Bolivar. At the time of its Davies Award application, the system included a 74-bed acute care hospital with a level 3 trauma center, five long-term care facilities with a total of 475 beds, one residential care facility with 60 beds, 16 rural physician clinics of which 11 were primary care certified rural health clinics, and home care services.

At the time of its award application, CMH had approximately 1,500 employees and 100 on-staff physicians, and provided care through approximately 130,000 clinic visits, 20,000 emergency department visits, 2,800 surgeries, a long-term care daily census of 423, and 14,500 home care visits on an annual basis.

MANAGEMENT

In 1999, CMH's strategic planning team questioned the ability of the organization's information systems infrastructure to support organizational objectives and strategies across the continuum of care.

As a result, the team initiated an information technology assessment and planning process, and developed, reviewed, accepted, and communicated a vision for Project Infocare. This project would involve implementation of an EHR and CPOE system across the system, and be used by 100 percent of admitting physicians and other caregivers.

Project Infocare had the following goals: to enable a patient to enter anywhere into the continuum of care and have a personal identity maintained across that continuum; to provide physicians and other caregivers access to all of the patient's medical information within the healthcare continuum; to ensure efficient and safe documentation by providers who were offered clinical decision support; and to enable technological advances in care in order to meet growing demands and offer new services.

An IS Steering Committee, including CMH's CEO, CIO, COO, director of finance, a physician champion, director of physician clinics, director of clinical services, and other clinical and non-clinical leaders, provided planning and implementation guidance.

Following a formal IT and systems assessment process, the IS Steering Committee recruited team members and led discussions to develop functional requirements for request for proposals (RFPs) from potential system vendors.

The system selection process was employee-driven and benefited from full administrative support. Thirty-nine project teams identified functional requirements for a new system (which resulted in a 200-page portion of the RFP), developed demonstration scenarios, participated in and evaluated demonstrations, conducted reference checks, participated in site visits, and recommended vendor(s) of choice. Their goal was to complete the RFP process and obtain signed contracts by December 2001.

MEDITECH, a vendor then with a 36-year history and use in more than 1,900 healthcare organizations, was recommended and selected as the primary vendor. The system also included a digital radiology PACS. The total budget for Project Infocare, which included software, hardware, personnel costs, travel, and training costs, was just more than $6 million. A ROI analysis indicated a positive return within five years of initial investment.

Implementation planning, conducted during a two-day off-site session using FranklinCovey's The 4 Roles of Leadership® model (pathfind, align, empower, model), created consensus on priorities.

CMH implemented Project Infocare in phases, including the following: kick off on March 2002; first applications (financial) in October 2002; core clinical applications by December 2002; paperless with full use of EHR and CPOE in the hospital by December 2003; and fifth and final long-term care facility live with CPOE by February 2005.

CMH used cross-departmental teams during implementation that were successful by giving equal loyalty to the project and their home departments. Two physician champions served as leaders of the medical staff for Project Infocare. Physician training was provided one-on-one and functionality, such as physician-specific orders sets, was personalized.

To transition to the new processes, CMH eliminated paper forms from the chart in phases. During the first phase, physicians were trained in e-signature, in entering daily notes, and in viewing test results and transcribed reports. At that point, the daily notes page, test results and transcribed reports were eliminated from the paper chart.

During the second phase, physicians were trained to enter procedure orders, and in the third phase to enter medication orders. During that time, other papers in the chart were transitioned to electronic format through the nursing documentation application, interfaces, or other applications.

On the date of implementation for the third phase (medication ordering), document scanning was also implemented to capture the remaining few paper documents and the paper charts were eliminated from the hospital.

Most data was collected through direct entry by physicians and caregivers. Other data was interfaced or scanned. IS specialists and super users provided support to physicians and other caregivers.

Each user received unique user names and passwords, and each user's access to the system was logged and audited. Access was limited both in which information within the EHR the user had access to and to which patients the user could see in the EHR. Staff members in physician clinics, for example, were allowed access only to the patients associated to their clinic physician. Billing personnel were allowed access only to demographic and billing information for patients. Physicians had access to all records and their use was audited.

FUNCTIONALITY

CMH targeted the elimination of paper in favor of query-able data and was seeking improvement in registration, scheduling, physician access to information, care delivery, care documentation, charge capture processes, and coordination of care across care settings.

CMH's strategy with regard to the medical record was to complete a comprehensive electronic record that would serve as an integrated, longitudinal health record across the continuum of care at CMH. At the time of the Davies Award application, CMH had created nearly 65,000 patient records within the Project Infocare EHR.

The EHR included all diagnostic test results and reports, physician notes and reports, orders, nursing and ancillary documentation, medication administration records, and patient demographics.

The records included an entry for all visits within the hospital, long-term care facilities, home care, and CMH physician clinics. Each patient had a unique EHR identification number that linked their visits and encounters together. The hospital EHR was the complete record and included all documentation of care; no paper charts were maintained. Any documentation not entered in a digital format was scanned and linked to the EHR for easy viewing.

The hospital and all long-term care facilities were wireless so physicians and caregivers were not "tethered to the wall" and could provide bedside documentation as appropriate for the setting and patients. CMH adopted a flexible approach to devices after learning of many unhappy hospitals that had invested large amounts in a single device type.

The EHR and CPOE provided decision support, including allergy and interaction checking, presentation of pertinent lab results, order specific rules, order sets, and knowledge bases.

The MEDITECH system offered more than 7,000 reports, including standardized, selection, custom, executive support, and other types of reports.

To enhance work flow and communications, data was immediately transferred within the system and available in all units and facilities. There was no need to copy records or re-enter data upon transfer.

The EHR system was fully integrated with financial and administrative applications, including general ledger, accounts payable, payroll/personnel, and materials management.

The system supported patient safety by eliminating handwriting/transcription errors, by requiring completeness of orders, through clinical decision support, and by providing access to clinical information and a patient's medical history.

System use was ubiquitous. In a one-hour sample from May 2, 2005, 115 users launched 1,260 requests to the EHR and information was delivered on 1,074 visits for 352 patients from eight different facilities. The EHR for the most popular patient in the hour was accessed by six different users from six different locations.

TECHNOLOGY

Prior to Project Infocare, CMH computing consisted of running limited financial and scheduling applications off green screens attached to an AS400. Dedicated 56-kilobyte (K) lines and terminal emulation provided limited remote access.

With Project Infocare, CMH added a network backbone and 50 IBM and HP servers to support networks connecting 33 buildings with wired and wireless access. Remote access was provided by Citrix Secure Gateway. More than 700 client workstations of the CMH network were a mixture of desktops, laptops, tablets, and mini laptops. More than 250 of these devices were mobile and communicated to the network via secure wireless.

The data model was a hierarchical, proprietary database from MEDITECH. The software structure allowed customization of processes and content through the tailoring of rules and master tables. Each data element was described in a data procedure module. Most could be accessed using a proprietary custom reporting tool. Additional custom fields or queries were specified by CMH and used for data collection, storage, and retrieval. CMH also built some rules that governed data entry.

Project Infocare met HIPAA requirements. CMH used HL7 interfaces for the data not directly entered into the EHR. The Project Infocare EHR was widely available on more than 700 devices in the 33 buildings connected to the CMH network and by remote access. Downtime planning, along with backup and data protection procedures safeguarded the EHR and ensured constant availability of patient care data.

VALUE

Since implementation of Project Infocare, CMH has already achieved many of the project's business ROI expectations. The system experienced an increase in adjusted occupied beds and in net patient revenue, a decrease in FTEs per adjusted occupied bed, and elimination of medical records scanning/microfilming costs.

In the area of process improvement, 92 percent of patients registered were known to the system and therefore not asked to repeat demographic information. Approximately 20,000 bar-coded express registration cards had been issued. More than one half of radiology exams were scheduled directly by a physician office.

Nearly 65,000 patient records had been created in the EHR. A unique EHR identification number linked visits together. Physicians were able to view individual visits, multiple visits, or all visits in one comprehensive online chart. More than $1 million in supply and procedure charges was captured per month as a by-product of care documentation. Yellow-sticker charging was eliminated from hospital inpatient floors.

CMH also experienced an improvement in the revenue cycle through a decrease in accounts receivable for the CMH physician clinics, an increase in supply charges per patient day, and a decrease in claim denials.

CMH indicated the next phases of Project Infocare would include full implementation of nursing and physician documentation and CPOE in the hospital emergency department, completion of implementation of clinical documentation in all CMH physician clinics, implementation of bar-coded bedside medication verification, enhanced physician documentation tools, enhanced clinical decision support, and a patient portal. "CMH is an enthusiastic supporter of the electronic health record vision," concluded the leadership team.

SECTION II

DAVIES AMBULATORY CARE
AWARD WINNERS

2003 DAVIES PRIMARY CARE AWARD WINNER
COOPER PEDIATRICS

ABOUT THE PRACTICE

Cooper Pediatrics is a one-site, solo practice located in Duluth, Georgia in the greater Atlanta area. Founded by Jeffrey D. Cooper, MD, FAAP, in 1992, Cooper employs a part-time physician's assistant, two part-time nurse practitioners, an office manager, a receptionist, an exit clerk, and three billing specialists. One part-time student assistant scans documents into the EHR.

At the time of its Davies Award application, Cooper Pediatrics served approximately 12,000 active patients, with Medicaid patients making up about 10 percent of the practice. The practice's services include well child care, immunizations, hearing screenings, vision screenings, minor injury management, sick visits, and daycare/school forms.

Cooper deployed an EHR on December 4, 1995. Eighteen months after going online, his office stored its paper charts off-site. Except for scanning and storing documents, Cooper Pediatrics was a paperless office.

MANAGEMENT

Cooper was not in the market for an EHR in 1995. However, after seeing a demonstration of a newly developed EHR, EncounterPRO® by JMJ Technologies of Atlanta, he decided to purchase and implement it in his office. With 3,500 active patients, at that time, Cooper Pediatrics was closed to new patients, so Cooper's business objectives were to open the practice to new patients and grow the business.

Cooper also defined specific objectives, including increased billings, revenues, profits, charges per visit, number of patient visits per day, patient volume, and staff, and decreased charting time, patient total wait time, drug refill time, and telephone call turnaround time.

Cooper's office manager was responsible for installation, the training schedule, and maintenance. The lead nurse was responsible for ongoing staff education on updates, training new staff members and reporting hardware and software issues.

FUNCTIONALITY AND IMPLEMENTATION

EncounterPRO, based on a work flow management system, allowed Cooper to customize and streamline collaboration among providers and staff in order to improve practice efficiency.

The EHR's data sets included problem lists, procedures, medical and nursing diagnosis, medication lists, allergies, demographics, diagnostic test results, radiology results, health maintenance alerts, and evaluation & management (E&M) coding. The clinical and patient narratives could be captured by free text, template-based text, dictation, or voice recognition.

The EHR provided results management, managing laboratory, radiology, and referral reports. It also kept track of tests for which no results had come back. The CPOE system encompassed electronic prescription writing, lab orders, x-ray orders, nursing entries (vitals screen), and referrals. All orders were highly configurable and could be part of the work flow. Buttons could be placed on any screen to order items automatically.

In the area of decision support, the EHR instantly calculated drug dosages based on weight, instantly plotted growth charts, and allowed for documentation of developmental milestones at well and/or sick visits. Tools included rules-based prompting with allergy alerts, immunization alerts, automatic screen sequencing, and note templates.

Patient support was provided through take-home reports that included all care instructions, a summary of all labs or tests ordered by the physicians, and a list of all medications and instructions.

The EHR fully integrated with GE Centricity, Cooper Pediatric's billing/scheduling system, which supplied information about appointments, schedules, and patient demographics. It also had a third-party interface showing the front office staff which specialists and labs were covered by what insurance companies. Reporting capabilities were extensive, including immunization tracking and other functions.

EncounterPRO, a client/server application, ran on Microsoft Windows® 2000 Server and Microsoft SQL Server™ 2000. The system evolved into a network featuring an upgraded Dell server and both thin and fat clients.

The user interfaces were akin to the touch screen-oriented systems in restaurants: one screen at a time, with only the most relevant data displayed and options presented.

Initial installation of a server, laboratory computer, and client servers in six exam rooms took about two days. Training of all practice staff took a total of four hours on a Saturday. The EHR was so easy to use the staff felt proficient within two weeks.

The practice took an incremental approach to converting the paper records. Little, if any, process redesign was needed to integrate the EHR due to its work-flow management approach, which automated the business processes according to the practice's way of doing business. Cooper Pediatrics did not have to change its routines to accommodate the EHR; it was configured to meet the practice's needs and preferences.

VALUE

After implementing the EHR on December 4, 1995 with 3,500 active patients, in January 1996, Cooper reopened his practice and added 600 new patients over the next six months. The practice continued to grow. By 1998, patient count reached 7,500 and by 2002, had grown to more than 12,000.

Annual gross billings increased 404 percent, from $490,000 in 1994 to $2,469,000 in 2002. Revenue increased 271 percent, from $419,700 to $1,557,300 in 2002. Cooper's revenue per full-time provider was 125 percent higher than the national norm.

Profit increased 102 percent from $15,900 in 1994 to $304,300 in 2002. Charges per visit increased 171 percent, from $50 in 1995 to $136 in 2002. Number of patient visits increased 62 percent, from 45 patients per day with two providers in 1995 to 73 patients per day with 3.25 providers.

Cooper Pediatrics totally eliminated chart pulls, going from 60 per day in 1995 to zero in 2002. Charting time decreased 75 percent, from an average of four minutes to less than one minute. No chart storage area was required and transcription costs were eliminated.

In terms of quality of care improvements, patient total wait time from check in to checkout decreased 42 percent, from one hour in 1995 to 35 minutes in 2002. Drug refill time and average telephone call turnaround time each decreased 75 percent, from one hour to 20 minutes or less. Patients were in and out of Cooper Pediatrics in 35 minutes. Immunization rates increased from 90 percent to 99 percent, and patient safety increased through legible, computer-generated prescriptions, allergy cross references, and other capabilities.

The original cost of the system in 1995 was $20,000 and through 2002, Cooper estimated he spent an additional $40,000 in upgrading and maintaining the system. The system paid for itself so quickly and generated so much additional income that Cooper was able to expand the office, moving to a larger facility with 11 exam rooms.

LESSONS LEARNED

Cooper cited the following factors as key to the EHR's success:
- Simultaneously accomplishing office tasks yields huge time savings. Everyone involved in the encounter saves time, effectively doubling and tripling the benefits.
- The automated work flow follows the physician's manual work flow; the processes were minimally re-engineered.
- Any re-engineering must simplify processes as much as possible.
- Dynamic short lists or templates are configurable to the preferences of each practice and to the preferences of each physician.
- Charting is easy to use. A long learning curve will doom a busy practice.
- The EHR system is quicker than paper at the point of use. The physician is the most expensive employee in the office and if he or she is taking longer to chart on the computer than on paper, the system will fail.

Among other things he wished he had known beforehand, Cooper cited: "Some computers are noisy. Terminal servers are quiet. A cartoon displayed on the touch screen helps to eliminate potential security issues." He stressed "time is the issue: Time is the only thing a physician has to sell. The EHR must save a physician time."

Cooper concluded as follows: "The IOM predicts that it will take seven years for most providers to migrate from paper records to a comprehensive EHR system. I disagree. More and more positive ROI data is finding its way into the journals. The bottom line is crystal clear: In terms of operating a small business, how can a physician afford not to automate the practice?"

2003 DAVIES PRIMARY CARE AWARD WINNER
EVANS MEDICAL GROUP

ABOUT THE PRACTICE

Evans Medical Group (EMG) is a four-physician primary care practice located in Evans, Georgia, outside of Augusta. Robert Lamberts, MD, senior partner, completed his residency at Indiana University Hospitals in Indianapolis, Indiana, and is board certified in Internal Medicine and Pediatrics.

During his residency, Lamberts was exposed to the work of Clement J. McDonald, MD, and the Regenstrief Medical Record System. Following training, Lamberts moved to Georgia, where he joined another physician in a practice owned by a hospital owned by Columbia/HCA, and then purchased back the practice.

MANAGEMENT

Given his experience with the Regenstrief system, investigating EHRs was one of the first things Lamberts pursued within his then two-physician independent practice. He looked at MedicaLogic, and agreed to purchase the company's new EHR, called Logician, and serve as a beta-test site for the training and installing of Logician by an arm of Blue Cross of Georgia. This organization saw the EHR as an opportunity to help manage care.

The cost of Logician to EMG was approximately $70,000, which Lamberts justified based on the expected increase in patient volume achievable through efficiencies offered by the EHR. EMG went live on Logician in July 1996.

The first version of Logician left little room for customization. Forms did not fit the practice's work flow, so EMG made templates on paper that pulled the data from the database and gave the staff the information needed during the visit. They would change information on the paper and have one of their assistants input the data at a later time.

MedicaLogic then offered a new Encounter Form Editor program, which gave users the tool for customizing the form templates.

EMG was truly a vanguard user. The practice attempted many ways to get information into the exam room and Lamberts finally decided in 1998 on using thin client terminals in the exam rooms over a Citrix platform. This would allow the practice to affect real-time decisions and use the computer, not as a record-keeping device, but as an interactive database.

Lamberts' small practice shot to the forefront of users of Logician, but making EHR work in a private-practice primary care office was difficult. As small business owners, physicians in private practice have to pay employees, bills, keep customers happy, and (hopefully) make a profit with an overhead in the region of 55 to 60 percent.

As EMG grew, the practice continued to increase its investment in both hardware and software. Lamberts and the office manager provided much of the practice's own technical support, installing new upgrades, and troubleshooting problems.

FUNCTIONALITY AND IMPLEMENTATION

EMG's EHR system ran on a mix of two-tiered fat clients and Citrix thin clients, all on an NT network. The practice moved back toward using laptop computers with wireless LAN as well as a trial with a Tablet PC workstation. An interface with the practice management system took demographics from this system and placed them into the EHR. The practice also interfaced with a major laboratory in the area, importing lab results as discreet data directly into the patients' database.

Encounter data was input into the chart via questionnaires filled out by the patient and input by the nurses, mainly using forms designed by Lamberts using the Encounter Form Editor.

Clinical information was also input by the clinician in the exam room, either by typing while the patient talked, using structured data (radio buttons, drop-down lists, etc.), or typing after the encounter.

If a patient required a medication, the physicians prescribed on Logician, printing out the prescription and giving it to the patient. If a consult was required, physicians sent a flag to the referral coordinator and she handled the referral process. Physicians used the orders feature on Logician when ordering lab or radiology tests.

Patient education was provided using handouts within Logician and handouts made by EMG staff. A custom form for phone calls that contained EMG's protocols as to how to handle various medical situations allowed nursing to handle a significant proportion of the phone calls without getting approval from the physician.

EMG's first attempt to measure and improve quality using the EHR involved targeting Pneumovax immunization in people over age 65. Through a simple search, EMG was able to increase immunization rates to more than 90 percent.

Childhood immunizations provided a good opportunity to measure and maximize outcomes, as well as increase business. The EHR allowed the practice not only to assure immunizations were up to date on patients who came to the office, but also to find those patients behind on immunizations. EMG regularly searched the database for all patients who were overdue for shots and alerted staff to call patients who were due for other well-care services. For example, EMG used the IHR to identify patients over age 65 in need of physical exams, diabetics without visits in the past 6 months, and hypertensive patients without visits in the past nine months.

EMG used disease management tools and forms designed by Clinical Content Consultants, LLC, for current care recommendations to guide care for the patient. EMG also used the tools for patient education.

VALUE

At the time of its Davies Award application, EMG was essentially paperless, and had not had specific charts made up for its patients since 1998. The practice expanded its EHR use consistently, despite significant provider turnover, increased patient volume, and periods of low cash flow. Buy in by both physicians and office staff significantly and consistently increased.

EMG used the EHR system to bring in more patients, and to improve the quality of patient care, and the practice's cash flow. Chart audits by insurance companies consistently gave EMG the highest grades possible and often effusive praise from the reviewer.

Patient volume continued to increase and satisfaction remained high. EMG increased profitability and income for primary care physicians in a time when incomes were decreasing.

LESSONS LEARNED

Lamberts offered the following lessons learned, which were relevant to the business in general and specific to the use of EHR:

- Invest in a system that will not become legacy. It is very important there be good support and an active user base. What is "hot" technology now will be out of date in a short time; so it is more important to find a company that will support the product rather than the specific features of the product.
- Find a company that allows customization of content. EMG worked hard at making forms fit its work flow, and did not have to adjust as much to the EHR as it had to adjust to the practice.
- Find a company that has a good product development cycle where feedback from users can be integrated quickly.
- Use "little bang" installation, which involves implementing only a small amount of the EHR at a time so the impact on work flow is minimal. Once the providers are given a tool and told not to use a lot of it, they generally are anxious to increase their adoption.
- Do not "force feed" changes, but rather first do it well yourself. If there is significant advantage to the change, demonstrate that advantage and adoption will be much less traumatic.
- Changes that may seem small often have a large trickle-down effect. Don't allow changes to happen unless you have discussed them and tried them in a smaller part of the practice to make sure there is not too great of an effect.
- Use the less enthusiastic users as your benchmark of adoption. It is easy to get adoption of enthusiasts, but if you can design tools that appeal to the least enthusiastic users, you will have much better success overall.

Lamberts concluded as follows: "To discuss EHR in our practice is to discuss our practice. Our computerized records are so central to our practice that it is impossible to think of our practice without them. They have clearly improved our work flow, patient volume, and quality. Using Logician, our practice has become a successful business in an era of increasing physician frustration."

2003 DAVIES PRIMARY CARE AWARD WINNER
ROSWELL PEDIATRIC CENTER

ABOUT THE PRACTICE

Started in 1978, Roswell Pediatric Center (RPC) has three independent practices located in the suburbs of North Atlanta, Georgia. Two of the practice locations are in Alpharetta, Georgia, and one is in Cumming, Georgia. Physical size ranges from 5,500 square feet to 7,000 square feet, with nine to 13 patient exam rooms in each location.

At the time of the Davies Award application, personnel included nine board-certified pediatricians, seven nurse practitioners, and approximately 60 other clinical and support staff. The combined three-site total number of annual patient visits was 82,000.

RPC's payor mix was 50 percent HMO contracts (including 20 percent capitation), 35 percent PPO contracts, 10 percent Medicaid, and 5 percent private pay. Nancy R. Babbitt, CMPE, is the practice administrator and served as the project manager for the practice's EHR planning and implementation.

MANAGEMENT

At its annual strategic planning retreat in December 2000, RPC's leaders targeted for improvement: universal access to the chart, quality of documentation, intra-office communication, work flow, and forms and referrals processing.

With 100 percent upfront physician acceptance, RPC's leaders made the decision to search and find a best-of-breed EHR product whose company was willing and able to develop an interface with RPC's then-current billing software (Promed).

A committee of three physicians and Babbitt screened EHR vendors with pediatric experience. They defined key elements of the EHR as progress notes, point-of-care coding and charge capture, physician order entry, prescription writing, and medical document imaging. Key selection factors included staff acceptance, functionality, flexibility, scalability, integration capability, company history and support availability, cost, and ROI.

The team selected NMS Medical Systems EHR software based on its intuitiveness and ease of use, ability to be customized, and efficiency. RPC purchased the system in August 2001 and told the vendor the practice's 80 employees in three locations needed to be live by flu season in November 2001, approximately 11 weeks later.

NMS provided a client services manager and a project manager to begin the planning, and RPC established a team of super users, which provided oversight for the input to NMS during the planning and implementation process. Physicians spent only a few hours a week reviewing documents during the planning stage, which lasted about three weeks.

During the first week, the team developed a 51-page project charter that outlined RPC's objectives and responsibilities and NMS responsibilities. This document served as the guiding force of the entire process and was a huge part of RPC's success in meeting its ambitious goals and 11-week time frame.

FUNCTIONALITY AND IMPLEMENTATION

NMS functionality included a three-screen approach to data entry. Virtually all documentation for an entire patient encounter was captured on only three screens through a point-and-click method, based on a template-driven system. RPC's clinical team and the NMS Medical Knowledge team developed the templates and customized these to match the practice's specific work flow and office patterns.

Ease of patient data retrieval and reformatting enabled the creation of reports, letters, forms, and graphs, whether for a single client record or the entire patient population. Customized decision support tools were available as was coding decision support. The latter was of particular interest given the intricacies of billing requirements. Use of such support resulted in fewer rejected claims and decreased administrative time spent on reconciliation.

NMS software provided automated charge capture functionality, with physician order entry generating appropriate charge details. On the front end, the practice management system communicated demographic and insurance information to the other products. On the back end, the EHR communicated billing information into the practice management system. NMS software also provided communication capability through the use of high priority alerts, bold text, and sticky notes.

With advice offered by IT consultants, RPC purchased 105 workstations, and decided to hardwire these. System implementation occurred in five phases:
- Planning (as already described);
- Familiarization during week one involved educating all staff and obtaining buy in;
- Configuration and verification in weeks two through six involved NMS team customization of visit outlines, care paths, order sets, reports, and document templates;
- Deployment during weeks seven and eight involved development of a system to enter patient history into the EHR; and
- Go live which occurred in week nine with 100 percent EHR use by the end of the second day.

To support the EHR's continued use, RPC had one staff member, a supervisor of IT, who spent 40 percent of her time working on clinical upgrades and changes.

VALUE

RPC experienced the following successes following EHR implementation: efficient reallocation of staff by streamlining communication to improve work flow, including turnaround time for triage calls, prescription refills (one hour to 20 minutes), and more efficient form and referral processing; significantly reduced chart pulls (from 440,000 per year to approximately 60,000 within 180 days); high parent and patient satisfaction due to ease of data access; decreased staff turnover, decreased claim denial rate; improved charge capture (by 18 percent); and short and efficient chart reviews.

The EHR cost RPC $53,700 per full-time clinician over five years or about $900 per clinician per month. This included the software maintenance, other software programs, ongoing IT expenses, and clinical upgrades.

The practice realized a positive ROI sooner than expected and was able to increase revenue through the reduction in the number of rejected claims. With medical necessity guidelines, the staff could select more specific ICD codes at the time of the encounter. The billing staff no longer had to spend time keying in codes or trying to interpret illegible handwriting, thus reducing necessary rework. This resulted in decreased costs through reduced time to process charge tickets, and reduced time to process rejected claims.

LESSONS LEARNED

At the initiation of the EHR project, RPC considered economic benefits secondary to the primary goals of improving intra-office work flow, communication, and patient care. If the magnitude of the ROI for improved charge capture had been recognized, RPC's leaders indicated the decision to purchase an EHR would have been made much sooner.

Other advice offered included the following:
- When evaluating EHRs, realize the physical layout of computer screens may affect usability. Make sure providers will use the system.
- A project charter that outlined every detail and everybody's responsibility helps to ensure implementation success.
- Consider buying uninterruptible power supply (UPS) capability for workstations in clinical areas instead of using plain surge protectors.
- Consider leasing the hardware instead of buying it. Leasing allows greater flexibility for additions, changes, and system upgrades.
- Involve an attorney and an experienced EHR consultant in negotiating vendor contracts and maintenance agreements.

Babbitt concludes, "Roswell Pediatric Center's 11-week EHR planning and installation was a success story. Staff and vendor alike dedicated substantial behind-the-scenes effort to planning, analysis and organization, and these were critical components of our success."

2004 DAVIES PRIMARY CARE AWARD WINNER
NORTH FULTON FAMILY MEDICINE

ABOUT THE PRACTICE

North Fulton Family Medicine is a two-site practice with offices in Alpharetta and Cumming, Georgia. The practice handles 51,000 patient encounters annually. At the time of its application, North Fulton had seven full-time physicians, nine nurse practitioners and physician assistants, and 38 additional clinical and administrative staff. Services included complete physical examinations, onsite x-rays, cardiac exercise stress testing, flexible sigmoidoscopy, pulmonary function testing, school and sports physicals, immunization updates, and worker's compensation examinations.

Three-quarters of North Fulton's patients are covered through managed care plans, 15 percent are insured through Medicare, and the remaining 10 percent are self-insured or covered under indemnity plans. The majority of North Fulton's patients are well educated and technologically savvy. Many work for leading technology companies in the rapidly growing suburbs Northeast of Atlanta where North Fulton's practice sites are located.

The Alpharetta office, with five physicians, handles more acute-care cases and has 30 exam rooms; the Cumming office, with two physicians, has 25 exam rooms.

MANAGEMENT

In 1997, North Fulton's service area was on the cusp of a population boom. The practice identified the need to add a satellite office to become accessible geographically to more patients, and to have enough space both to accommodate new patients and to maximize same-day encounters when the numbers increased.

Prior to implementing its EHR solution, North Fulton had four physicians treating 13,000 patients. The practice identified numerous opportunities to recoup the time and money spent on administrative functions, and to improve the quality of patient care while growing the practice. In particular, the practice sought to save cost spent on additional FTEs, supplies, and chart storage space. The practice also knew it lost reimbursement due to miscoded procedures and charges.

Ultimately, the North Fulton's leaders felt an EHR along with work flow improvements and upgraded telephone systems were the best avenues for working toward the practice's overall growth strategy while simultaneously reducing overhead and improving patient care.

Dr. Thomas E. Bat, the practice leader, and Dr. James R. Morrow led the improvement effort at North Fulton. Together, they researched EHR solutions and worked to get buy in from other practice physicians and staff.

FUNCTIONALITY AND IMPLEMENTATION

After a seven-month search and many site visits, North Fulton selected A[4] Health Systems'® HealthMatics EMR Electronic Medical Record and later interfaced it with HealthMatics Ntierprise Practice Management System. To further expand its system's capabilities, the practice also used TeleVox Lab Calls to report patient lab results, HealthMatics Assure to enhance patient record safety, and recently implemented HealthMatics Access, promoting e-communication between patients and the practice.

The implementation plan and training was executed by Dr. Bat and Dr. Morrow in cooperation with the EHR's vendor implementation specialists. Each exam room was equipped with a desktop computer where care providers were able to access patient charts and enter information at the patient's bedside.

The EHR organized communication and chart information within the practice and with outside practitioners. It managed orders, procedures, prescriptions, laboratory results and other data previously collated into patient charts by hand onto paper. The solution enabled North Fulton to maintain problem and medication lists; generate preventative care reminders; receive medication interaction, allergy or lab abnormality alerts; and harvest patient information to generate population-based reports.

Prescriptions, referrals and orders were generated automatically, again reducing hassles for the patient. Physicians were able to log on from home via secure high-speed Internet for decision support while on call as well as to manage the practice while out of the office.

The entire system was password protected and programmed for automatic time-outs, increasing security of information. Data access was restricted depending on need within the practice. Additionally, North Fulton used HealthMatics Assure disaster recovery, enabling backup of all information on remote servers, facilitating security of patient records, and allowing the practice to meet 2005 HIPAA guidelines.

The EHR interfaced with all major lab information and messaging systems, as well as Midmark Diagnostics.

Core functions included the following: history and physical (the EHR used the simple object access protocol (SOAP) format); visit notes, which could be customized and templates for protocols were provided upfront; problem list; and medications.

North Fulton created medication lists for each physician and for the entire practice, making medication selection a simple point-and-click procedure. Electronic prescriptions could be managed via fax and e-mail directly from the chart, greatly reducing chart handling and refill turnaround times.

Drawing from the incorporated Medispan® drug database, the EHR also sent critical warnings. Radiology reports could be input directly into the EHR and were simplified.

Other core functions included:

- Lab results (bidirectional communication enabled labs to be ordered from the point of care and the results to be delivered to providers' desktops where an alert signaled abnormal results);
- Reports and correspondence from outside the practice; and
- Practice-based analysis that allowed physicians to: identify at-risk patient populations [i.e. run a report to find all patients on a medication recalled by the Food & Drug

Administration (FDA)], use the database for disease management, clinical trials and tracking patients patterns, compare patients with similar conditions and treatment plans, support routine health maintenance with automated reminders, and evaluate practice compliance with HEDIS requirements.

North Fulton implemented the EHR on December 17, 1998. The process involved significant onsite and off-site work to establish required clinical customizations, link the two practice sites, and train key users and the entire employee population.

It took two to three patient visits to get the electronic chart fully populated with patient information, but the practice did not lose productivity. North Fulton was able immediately to treat 15 scheduled patients per provider each day, as well as 70 to 75 walk-ins or same-day appointments.

VALUE

At the time of the Davies Award, seven physicians, one nurse practitioner, eight physician assistants, and 20 nursing assistants used the EHR solutions to handle 51,000 patient encounters annually. The EHR enabled North Fulton to become more efficient and expand to meet demand. In fact, the physicians and staff refer to the practice as "the house that the EHR built."

After EHR implementation, the practice size literally exploded, growing from four to 14 providers and from 15 to 55 exam rooms in five short years.

Value highlights included the following:
- Two front-office staff processed 100 patients per day in 1998; five years later, it processed more than 330 patients per day.
- Recouped transcription costs since implementation totaled approximately $775,000.
- Time on administrative functions drastically decreased: chart handling time per day decreased from 625 minutes to zero; missing chart searches time per day decreased from 330 minutes to zero; transcription processing time per day decreased from 705 minutes to zero; and lab result handling time per day decreased from 570 minutes to zero.
- With EHR and LabCalls, the practice reduced the load on its overtaxed phone system by nearly 32 percent.
- First year results revealed the practice's growth strategy resulted in an estimated savings of $4,594 per day or $1,249,568 annually; ongoing annual savings of $275,000 on average were expected.

LESSONS LEARNED

The primary lesson learned, according to Dr. Morrow, was, "The sooner you implement an EHR system, the better off you will be. Once you implement a system you'll never want to go back to paper, but a key piece of the puzzle is to get the buy in from all of the physicians from the very beginning.

Other advice offered by North Fulton's leaders includes:
- Be proactive with technology solutions instead of reactive. Continuously identify tools and solutions that can help grow the practice. This makes growth much less painful and less expensive.

- Look to the future. Consider your expected growth and determine what solution will best fit your current needs as well as those you see on the horizon.
- Ensure the EHR vendor is a forward-thinking partner, and one with sufficiently robust products and support services to enable the practice to achieve its goals.

The practices leaders conclude, "In North Fulton's case, the time spent researching EHRs and going on site visits was invaluable in selecting a vendor they felt confident would—and continue to—help meet practice business and patient care goals through innovative solutions."

2004 DAVIES PRIMARY CARE AWARD WINNER
OLD HARDING PEDIATRIC ASSOCIATES

ABOUT THE PRACTICE

Old Harding Pediatric Associates is a 14-physician, two-site pediatric practice located in the greater Nashville, Tennessee area. In the year it won the Davies Award, the practice employed 32 FTE nurses and 27.5 FTE additional staff, had approximately 400 visits per day and 72,500 patient encounters each year, and cared for 23,000 patients.

The primary clinic is open seven days a week, including nighttime clinic hours Monday through Friday. The satellite clinic is open five days a week for daytime hours. Both offices have moderately complex laboratories managed by medical technicians who perform approximately 230 labs between both sites.

MANAGEMENT

Old Harding Pediatrics' primary goal in implementing an EHR was to improve the quality of patient care and to continue to provide excellent care during implementation. If this goal could be achieved, the practice expected also to improve physician and office staff efficiency, improve patient satisfaction, and increase office profitability.

Old Harding Pediatrics defined specific quality improvement targets, including having complete, legible medical records available upon arrival of every patient, and ready assistance with clinical decision-making. The practice considered automated alerts for drug allergies or medications that were incompatible to be essential.

To improve physician and staff efficiency, the practice wanted to reduce the need for shadow charts held by both clinics. In addition to other goals, Old Harding Pediatrics wanted to improve communication between all departments, decrease turnaround time for triage calls, prescriptions, and referrals, and improve patient satisfaction. Office profitability would be enhanced by having a more accurate method of documenting appropriate coding levels for visits.

The EHR selection and implementation team included a physician (implementation clinical lead), nurse (implementation lead), executive administrator (project manager), and an assistant administrator (implementation administrative lead). The practice contracted with an outside source for an implementation technical lead, who worked with the practice's engineering services analyst to fully assess and plan for the implementation.

Following a strategic planning effort in 2001 that identified the need for an EHR, the team began researching software companies, defining product and vendor criteria, and reviewing potential products. The team selected an EHR system offered by Cleveland, Ohio-based Noteworthy Medical Systems that met the criteria, which included looking as close to a paper chart as possible and being easy to learn and use.

FUNCTIONALITY AND IMPLEMENTATION

Core functions of the EHR system were intuitive. The well child or illness reason drove history and physical exam questions for the visit chosen by the nurse. The majority of information could be captured by selecting from pick lists, but information could also be entered as free text, if necessary.

The problem list was visible on the summary page when a patient chart was opened and this page included current medications and allergies. Radiology exams could be ordered in the system and a synopsis of results entered manually when the report came into the office. Referrals could be ordered within the system by the physician and a report run by referral staff to facilitate complete authorizations and prior approvals for referred patients. The EHR included laboratory ordering and results reporting functionality, and offered an extensive pediatric medical knowledge base that provided a springboard for physician customization.

The software ran on one main server with client software loaded on each exam's station or physician's station. The client software requested data from the server delivering real-time information. Only data related to the current patient were local to the client, but then updated back to the server. An imaging component within the EHR scanned and stored the images to a SQL Server.

Noteworthy's EHR employed a simple, comprehensive interface to generate and transmit charge capture information. The back-office, including scheduling and billing, was accomplished through Computer Science Corporation's MDR portal that was presented to the user within Internet Explorer.

The entire network infrastructure was based on Microsoft Windows 2000 network operating system. Each client had Windows XP allowing a very graphical interface use with patients.

Old Harding Pediatrics' implementation process consisted of seven main focus areas: project charter, work flow assessment, medical knowledge configuration, hardware considerations, EHR and practice management system interface, paper chart transition, and staff training and encouragement.

Throughout the planning and implementation phases, staff had opportunities to become familiar with the system by using one of two training environments set up in the offices. Two super users were educated at Noteworthy's headquarters where they prepared to serve as clinical and administrative leads for the project. During the week of go live with the EHR every staff member was given intensive hands on training by members of both implementation teams.

Physician practice style was changed greatly by removing a paper chart from the patient room. The senior physician, who served as executive sponsor for the project, showed excitement and readiness for the changes about to take place. His optimism spread throughout the other physicians and staff.

Old Harding Pediatrics achieved 100 percent use of the EHR by day four of use. Many physicians had stopped with paper charts on day two and all had stopped by day four. Every patient check in, triage call, sick visit, well child visit, nurse visit, lab entry, and billing procedure was documented in the EHR by the end of that same week.

All prescriptions were generated electronically and given to patients. SOAP notes were printed often for use with referrals and visits to the emergency room. Chronic illness summary reports were routinely sent with all referrals. The practice eliminated the need to handwrite such reports. Every patient seen for a physical received a physical exam report with growth information and percentiles listed. Vaccine information sheets printed at sign out if a vaccine had been administered. The summary page contained a section for wellness rules that listed immunizations needed, suggested referrals, and suggested labs.

VALUE

Old Harding Pediatrics defined EHR implementation success as improving quality of patient care, achieving 100 percent staff acceptance, using the EHR for 100 percent of patient encounters by the end of the first week, and having a virtually paperless office by the end of the first year. The practice achieved these goals.

Continuity of care between both offices was excellent because the practice was able to eliminate lag time between information traveling between the two offices. Patients were excited about the change and looked forward to getting their printed Physical Exam reports and educational handouts. Triage nurses no longer had to search for charts and turnaround time for callback had been markedly reduced. Prescriptions were always legible and the practice eliminated callbacks from pharmacies to verify information. Papers were not lost in the filing system, because once they were read, they were instantly scanned into patient charts. Charges were captured efficiently and reimbursement times lessened. Finally, Old Harding Pediatrics' report tracking enabled the practice to analyze both clinical and administrative data that were useful when developing policies and protocols.

LESSONS LEARNED

As with any change, areas of adjustment were required. Paper chart transition became a much more detailed task than first thought. Before charts were sent to storage, data had to be entered and then verified by a nurse, and signed off by a physician. Staff roles evolved from filing and copying to data entry and scanning. Policies and procedures had to incorporate EHR-specific rules. Practice styles were altered for physicians, because they had computers in rooms instead of charts. But because of in-depth research on hardware, the computers did not come in between the physician and the patient.

Ultimately, Old Harding Pediatrics credits its success with implementation to physician buy in for the product. Noteworthy offered an EHR that looked similar to a chart and was therefore, less daunting to all of the practice's users. All physicians had some level of apprehension about such a monumental change of practice style, but they could also see the benefits that connecting with the electronic world would have on the care provided for children.

Old Harding Pediatrics' leaders conclude: "What once seemed like an impossibility for us has now become an extraordinary way to care for and educate our patients while receiving swift and accurate reimbursement."

2004 DAVIES PRIMARY CARE AWARD WINNER
PEDIATRICS AT THE BASIN

ABOUT THE PRACTICE

Pediatrics at the Basin is a two-physician private pediatric practice located in Pittsford, New York, a suburb of Rochester. Alice Loveys, MD, and Janet Cranshaw, MD, opened the practice in 2002, and in 2004, the year their practice won the Davies Award, had a staff of approximately three FTEs and provided 4,200 annual patient encounters. Ninety-five percent of the practice's patients belong to an HMO.

MANAGEMENT

As working mothers of young children, Drs. Loveys and Cranshaw were motivated to implement an EHR more for personal reasons than financial reasons. They both left high-volume, paper chart-based practices where "there was never enough time to adequately evaluate patients, document the care given, and provide detailed enough instructions for care to the patients."

With objectives that included wanting to achieve a better balance of home and professional life, to create an office with an unrushed atmosphere, and to provide thorough medical care, Loveys, Cranshaw, and a member of a local sister office, Greg Meyer, reviewed several EHR systems before selecting SOAPware by Docs Inc., a Fayetteville, Arkansas-based company.

Selection criteria included the company's reputation, software licensing and support costs, hardware and hardware support costs and requirements, customizability, further development plans and upgrade costs, and available modules and interfaces.

Initial cost for EHR software was $1,500 per physician with $300 per year per physician in ongoing cost for technical support and upgrades. The practice's initial hardware investment was $10,000, with ongoing cost of $1,500 per year.

FUNCTIONALITY AND IMPLEMENTATION

The EHR's technical infrastructure was based on Microsoft Access. The office had a hardwired network with a Linux server and the exam rooms, physicians' desk, nurses' station, front desk, and billing desk were equipped with a PC with high-speed Internet access.

The EHR offered several modules for interfaces with a variety of products, including practice management systems, local laboratories, spirometers, EKG machines, and other data collection tools. Pediatrics at the Basin interfaced with the local laboratory, ACM, using an HL7 interface program as well as a file transfer protocol (FTP) program to receive results directly into the patients' charts. The local lab provided support for its part of the interface and the EHR vendor provided support for the development of this specific interface.

SOAPware featured pre-written templates for many common types of encounters. Templates provided a framework for history, physical, assessments, and plans with quick, easy-to-select toggle switches to record positives and negatives.

Pediatrics at the Basin was able to easily modify these templates or create new templates to meet the practice's needs. Nurses chose a template for common encounters: well child visits, common illness and injury visits, phone calls, and medication refills. More detailed history and physical could be entered and modified with the keyboard, but the templates saved time and duplicated effort by the provider.

Other functionality included the following:

- Medications could be compared with allergies and other medications to identify potential drug interactions or allergic reactions.
- Radiology reports and outside correspondence, such as referral letters and emergency visits, could be scanned into the report section of the chart.
- Results from the laboratory could be entered directly into the patient chart via a computer interface installed by the practice. New results appeared on a to-do list so staff members were alerted to new results as soon as they were available.
- One-click printing of a personal medical history (problem list, medications, family history, allergies, etc.), and instructions for care and follow up at illness visits enabled the practice to provide information to the patient or family at each yearly physical exam and illness visits.
- Routine preventive care and health maintenance items, such as screening for lead exposure, diabetic care follow up, and cholesterol screening, could be identified. Each time the patient's chart was opened a reminder alert would come on the screen.
- The interface to billing enabled providers to generate a super bill from the patient encounter.

Full conversion from a paper-based system to the SOAPware EHR took the practice about a year.

VALUE

Pediatrics at the Basin fully succeeded in meeting its objectives for the EHR. Significant work flow changes positively impacted the physicians' face-to-face patient time and they were able to more completely and accurately record patient encounters, making this information legible for retrieval by other healthcare providers.

The application of clinical information provides the best example of the EHR's value. The practice used clinical guidelines provided by the Rochester Health Commission to create templates for the initial evaluation and follow-up care of patient with asthma, for example. The practice's assessment was supported by the history and physical, and how treatment was directed in accordance with national guidelines. The template could be easily modified as recommendations were updated.

The EHR also assured information in the chart was current, accurate, and immediately available upon the patient's arrival at the practice or during a telephone call. The EHR greatly enhanced efficiency at Pediatrics at the Basin, lowering the overall cost of healthcare and leaving the practitioners more time for other commitments. The practice experienced significant improvement in patient care as a result of the automated asthma action plan, which, based on guidelines as described earlier, outlined exactly what actions or treatments the parents or child should follow, depending on specific conditions or symptoms.

Ongoing savings or revenue increases were estimated to be $16,800 per year for charting/pulled charts, $1,000 to $1,400 per year for new patient entry, $10,000 per year for transcription expenses not incurred, and $20,000 to $30,000 for office personnel.

Time available for patient encounters increased from 10 minutes per acute and 20 minutes per well child visit to 15 minutes per acute and 30 minutes per well child visit. Pharmacy callback time decreased from 15 minutes per call to 3 minutes per call.

LESSONS LEARNED

Pediatrics at the Basin cited "a good team to select, implement and make the most of EHR system, and an excellent IT person as part of the team" as critical success factors. The practice advised other practices that EHR selection and implementation should be a gradual process, and to investigate what functions are important in a system to the particular office's work flow before purchasing a system.

The physicians concluded: "Offices should give themselves time to select and implement a system and build in some time for a team member to develop customizations. The time invested will be well worth it and you'll be able to enjoy all the benefits an EHR offers professionally and personally."

2004 DAVIES PRIMARY CARE AWARD WINNER
RIVERPOINT PEDIATRICS

ABOUT THE PRACTICE

Riverpoint Pediatrics is a single-site solo practice located in the Lakeview area of Chicago, Illinois. Founded in 1978 by Armand A. Gonzalzles, MD, FAAP, the practice employs four full-time-equivalent staff. At the time it won the Davies Award, Riverpoint Pediatrics had nearly 7,000 annual patient encounters and served 5,800 active patients, 20 percent of whom were enrolled in HMOs.

Riverpoint Pediatrics' services include well child care, immunizations, tympanometry, vision screening, minor injury evaluation and management, sick visits, school, preschool and disability forms, and family leave forms. The practice also gives nebulized aerosol treatments.

Gonzalzles deployed an EHR at Riverpoint Pediatrics on January 9, 2000.

MANAGEMENT

Gonzalzles' interests in using an EHR in his practice dated to the 1980s, but cost, integration with practice management systems, and ease-of-use barriers made EHR purchase and use prohibitive. After buying back his practice from a multi-specialty hospital managed group in 1999, Gonzalzles found an efficient, affordable EHR—EncounterPRO developed by JMJ Technologies of Atlanta, Georgia—in November 1999, and the software was installed in his practice two months later.

Gonzalzles' primary business objective in EHR implementation was to increase the quality of patient care by spending more time with patients and less time documenting. Other objectives were to increase revenues, physician profit, charges per visit, number of patients visits per day, patient volume, immunization rate, collection rate, and managed care reimbursement, and decrease claims denied due to coding errors, insurance turnaround time, charting time, patient waiting time, drug refill time, and telephone turnaround time. Gonzalzles also wanted to track total operating cost as percent of medical revenue, make more productive use of charting space, eliminate chart pulls and transcription cost, and expand office space.

FUNCTIONALITY AND IMPLEMENTATION

Gonzalzles assumed responsibility for hardware and software installation, and his office manager assumed responsibility for the training schedule. The lead medical office assistant was responsible for ongoing staff education on updates, training new staff members, and reporting hardware and software issues.

EncounterPro offered Gonzalzles both a work flow system and a full-fledged work flow management system. The work flow management system created, executed, monitored, and edited the practice's work flow system to reflect the practice's clinical needs, personal preferences, and business requirements.

Intended users for the EHR included physicians, nurses, and all staff members. In addition, insurance and managed care plan auditors could be given a temporary password for access to medical records.

Core functions of the EHR included history and physicals, visit notes, problem list, medications, radiology reports, reports and correspondence from outside the practice, laboratory results, patient support, and internal reports.

Clinical decision support tools in routine use included integrated and aggregated displays of patient data either one visit at a time or in summary. Problem lists, immunization records, medication lists, and allergies to food, drugs or other were displayed. Allergy alerts fed from allergy input and flashed a warning when a drug the patient was allergic to was chosen. Immunization alerts showed on the opening screen of each chart along with a digital picture of the child.

The EHR was integrated with Riverpoint Pediatrics' practice management system, Lytec, and interfaced with other practice management systems. EncounterPro was a client/server application that ran on Microsoft Windows 2000 or 2003 Server and Microsoft SQL Server 2000. The EHR used touch screen monitor systems and Tablet PCs. The examination, subjective, objective, assessment and plan were done by touch, and the chart was signed off by use of an electronic signature pad. Paper in the form of laboratory, consultations, x-ray, and other reports were scanned into the EHR and attached to the appropriate chart.

Gonzalzles performed the network management work himself and hired a local technician for some tasks. The practice started with an IBM Netfinity server and upgraded the CPU from 512RAM to 1GB, and went from two 18GB drives to four with dual processors. The practice also went from fat to thin clients and exchanged its router for a switch, which increased speed tenfold.

On installation of the EHR, Gonzalzles immediately began using the EHR to chart all patient encounters, but chose not to scan in all of the existing paper charts. He brought the paper chart into the exam room for the first few months, but stopped that practice within about six months. The staff charted chronic illnesses so they could leave the paper chart on the shelf if the patient had already had at least one encounter charted in the EHR. The staff also keyed in the vaccine histories. Staff later moved the paper charts off-site to free up more floor space.

Riverpoint Pediatrics' staff and Gonzalzles were originally trained during a single week of onsite training. Gonzalzles continued to chart patients on paper for the first two days, and then charted every patient on the EHR beginning the third day of training.

VALUE

Following implementation of the EHR, Riverpoint Pediatrics experienced vast improvements in patient care, collections, and insurance audits. Gonzalzles was able to spend more time with patients, thus meeting his primary business objective for the EHR.

Following implementation of the EHR, the practice increased revenue more than 77 percent and profit nearly 91 percent, increased charges per visit almost 50 percent (from $56 per encounter in 1999 to $78 per encounter in 2003), increased by 50 percent the number of patient visits per day, increased patient volume from 2,200 in 1999 to 4,400 in 2004, increased immunization rates from 50 percent to 95 percent, and increased the collection rate from 52 percent to 88 percent.

Riverpoint Pediatrics also decreased the number of claims denied due to coding and other errors to zero, decreased insurance turnaround time from 30 to 60 days to an average of 15 days, decreased charting time from 30 to 60 minutes to 10 to 15 minutes, decreased patient wait time from an hour or more to 36 minutes, decreased drug refill time from 24 to 48 hours to 15 minutes, and decreased telephone call turnaround time from 24 hours or more to less than 15 minutes.

Post EHR implementation, the practice also eliminated chart pulls, the chart storage area, transcription cost, expanded office space, and enhanced physician satisfaction and customer service. Quality review scores increased from 65 percent to 95 percent, and medication errors were vastly reduced or eliminated.

Many of Gonzalzles' processes were easily engineered into the EHR, so he and his staff were able to conduct business without altering the efficient processes they had developed. The leased EHR system, with initial costs for hardware at $18,500, software at $7,000, and installation at $1,300, paid for itself in three years.

LESSONS LEARNED

Gonzalzles noted the ability to see a patient, code the visit, and transmit the bill almost instantaneously "is invaluable in today's managed care market. It is no longer a matter of volume, but rather a matter of working smarter in this environment." As other critical success factors, he cited the fact the EHR's automated work flow followed his training, charting must be easy and fun, and the EHR must be faster than paper entry, especially at the point of use.

Gonzalzles offered the following words of advice:

- System administrators come with all levels of certification. Cisco and Microsoft certifications are most important when relying on someone to set up a network and install software.
- Learn the basics of hardware and software maintenance.
- Some computers are better then others. Stick with name brands that are tried and true.
- Make sure you have two or three backup systems to save data and programs on a daily basis. Check your backup and restore capabilities on a regular basis.
- Use security on your workstations; a screensaver will suffice with an alpha numeric password access.

He concluded with the following remarks: "The physician needs both an EHR and a practice management system to run a viable practice. Pediatrics and other primary care specialties are no longer volume businesses. We must work smarter, code better, and chart in compliance with what the physician hospital organization (PHO) dictates. The EHR has made it possible for this practice to take on a 'concierge' approach to solo practice rather then a volume approach. The EHR changed my outlook on pediatric practice and has made it possible for me to evolve in this era of managed care, shrinking reimbursements, and smaller patient volumes."

2005 DAVIES PRIMARY CARE AWARD WINNER
SOUTHEAST TEXAS MEDICAL ASSOCIATES, LLP

ABOUT THE PRACTICE

Southeast Texas Medical Associates, LLP (SETMA), is a 24-physician practice in Beaumont, Texas, a city of 115,000 located approximately 90 miles Northeast of Houston, Texas. Originating in 1995 as a single location, primary care practice with five providers, SETMA quickly evolved into an integrated delivery system with three clinical locations. By 2004 at the time of its Davies Award application, it employed 272 personnel, including 12 nurse practitioners, and had a patient base of more than 80,000 patients.

SETMA provides a full range of primary care services and is supported by specialists in many specialties and subspecialties. In addition, the organization has separate locations for billing, physical therapy, hospice, home health, and mobile x-ray, and operates a level two, moderately complex reference laboratory. Annual patient encounters for all services were approximately 263,000 in 2004.

MANAGEMENT

SETMA's partners realized the pursuit of excellence in clinical care required EHR, and the complexities of 21st century medicine required data management rather than document management.

SETMA's specific clinical and business objectives for an EHR included improved quality of care, improved patient safety, comprehensive clinical documentation, increased work flow efficiencies, increased reporting efficiencies, and increased physician productivity and satisfaction.

Believing its future growth was limited by the paper-based medical record, in 1998 SETMA purchased EHR and electronic practice management (EPM) systems from NextGen™ Healthcare Information Services.

The criteria for selecting the vendor and products included the financial stability of the vendor and its commitment to research and development; availability of support and the company's reputation among existing customers; product scalability and flexibility; the ability to transition from paper to electronic documentation with the lowest possible interference with patient care and without impeding physicians' abilities to deliver quality care; and the ability for successful interaction between the EHR, practice management system, laboratory information systems, scanning solutions, office software, and a number of other functions.

FUNCTIONALITY AND IMPLEMENTATION

After extensive development of a unique database between April 1998 and December 1998, SETMA went live with the EHR on January 22, 1999, with one pod at a time.

A pod is a self-contained clinical staff team comprised of physicians, nurses, nurse practitioners, and unit clerks. SETMA took additional pods live on the EHR within the next months, and was seeing all patients using the EHR by February 26, 1999.

The EHR was available across the entire network, providing secure access to patient data at all points of service, including emergency rooms, three hospitals, all clinical locations, providers' residences, and nursing homes. All staff used the EHR. All databases ran on Microsoft SQL Server 2000 sp3. Then-current hardware included 22 IBM xSeries360 servers in an active/passive cluster.

Through template-driven algorithms and using point-and-click, voice-activate data capture, typing and/or scanning, healthcare providers could capture history and physical, visit notes, problem list, medications, radiology reports, reports and correspondence from outside the practice, and laboratory results. EHR implementation provided documentation of more than 260,000 patient encounters, 672,000 incoming telephone calls, 15,000 x-rays, and 4,000 EKGs each year, as well as documentation of all nursing home patient visits, physical therapy visits, and other functions.

SETMA's implementation also resulted in the practice's ability to fax all prescriptions to pharmacies, communicate via e-mail and e-mail laboratory results to patients with patient authorization and when proper security is in place on both ends of the transaction, and receive requests for appointments, referrals, billing information, or laboratory data via SETMA's Web site, among many other capabilities.

VALUE

SETMA reached and exceeded all of its expectations in purchasing the EHR. In addition the practice transitioned from an EHR to EPM, which increased the value of the EHR by providing increased quality of care, increased patient safety, decreased costs, improved patient/provider communications, and improved ability to evaluate provider performance.

As documentation of improved quality of care, SETMA indicates, among other improvements, prior to implementing the EHR, the practice had a 20 percent immunization compliance rate; post EHR, the rate exceeded 80 percent. SETMA was able to establish disease-specific clinics for diabetes, lipid management, and six other common clinical conditions that were supported by template-driven, national standards of care, disease-specific management tools.

In the area of increased work flow efficiencies, as another example, SETMA indicated the EHR helped to improve prescription processes, streamline referral management, enable online communication, improve response time to patient inquiries, improve the drug recall process, and improve inquiry documentation.

Financial benefits included increased income due to the electronic superbill (the overall average charge per patient visit increased to $206 from $171 and the average collection increased to $104 from $80), increased revenue (by nearly $3 million annually), reduced chart costs (resulting in annual savings of more than $22,000), reduced transcription costs (with annual savings of more than $340,000), increased billable charges (more than $150,000 in billable charges), reduced supplies costs (more than $380,000 in paper and supply costs), reduced chart staff, and decreased claim denials.

LESSONS LEARNED

SETMA's leaders indicated if a practice is to be successful in implementing EHR, the practice will, for a brief time, give more attention to the EHR than it seems to be giving to patients. After the implementation process, however, "high tech" will promote "high touch."

SETMA's leaders caution other practices to fully use the strengths and capacities of the EHR. "If the EHR is only a glorified transcription machine, it isn't worth it," they note. The practice of medicine and healthcare delivery are so complicated today they require systems solutions to accomplish such tasks as monitoring the behavior of patients, examining patterns of behavior among the providers, and affecting the health of a population of people, they observe.

If an organization is going to successfully implement an EHR, there has to be a champion who is respected by most of the providers, a vendor with a sound financial position and a proven track record for successful implementation, support and continued product development, adequate support staff both managerial and technological, adequate preparation and training, and commitment to a final schedule for implementation.

SETMA's leaders conclude: "Perhaps the greatest lesson we learned was that it is never either too late or too early to start implementing a system. Now is the time to get started. The hurdle is significant, but once surmounted the benefits are enormous to the patient, to the provider, to the practice, to the payors and to the public."

2005 DAVIES PRIMARY CARE AWARD WINNER
SPORTS MEDICINE &
ORTHOPEDIC SPECIALISTS, PC

ABOUT THE PRACTICE

Sports Medicine & Orthopedic Specialists (SMOS) is a four-physician practice that specializes in the care of athletes and care of injuries in an active population in Birmingham, Alabama. At the time it won the Davies Award, SMOS had 20,000 annual patient encounters and employed a clinical staff of nine and an administrative staff of six.

Serving a metropolitan area with a population of slightly more than 1 million, the practice's physicians are the team physicians for the local professional arena football league and for 20 high schools and middle schools in the area. SMOS also has a large referral base of area primary care physicians and former patients. The practice mix is approximately 50 percent sports medicine and 50 percent general orthopedics.

MANAGEMENT

In early 2002, it was evident to the practice's physicians, and clinical and administrative staff that, with the rapid growth of the new practice, medical records and charts were becoming a major challenge. Samuel Goldstein, who founded the practice as Baptist Sports Medicine and Orthopedics Specialists in 2000, began to research and evaluate EHR systems. At that time, the practice had two physicians and seven clinical and support staff.

Criteria for an EHR system included the following: applicability of the system to the specialty of orthopedic surgery and sports medicine; cost of initial system investment; ability to eliminate transcription cost; availability of charts and physician access to the charts at home; simultaneous access to the record by multiple users; ability to increase office efficiency; and ability to respond promptly to referring physicians.

After review of numerous systems, SMOS selected AllMeds from the AllMeds Company, headquartered in Oak Ridge, Tennessee. SMOS implemented AllMeds in September 2003. Dr. Goldstein, Cherie Miner, MD, and the registered nurse, Denise Godstein, were responsible for clinical implementation and patient flow organization during the transition to an EHR. The business manager and billing clerk were responsible for the administrative side of the transition. AllMeds Company provided support to make the EHR work at SMOS.

FUNCTIONALITY AND IMPLEMENTATION

The AllMeds program was a template-driven system, but also offered limited free-form typing or dictation functionality. The program was based on the familiar SOAP note format. The system could track CPT codes performed and ordered in the office, and help ensure coding compliance by tracking information bullet points that gave the practitioner a suggested visit CPT code.

Notes to referring physicians, physical therapy orders, and orders for Magnetic Resonance Imaging (MRIs) and other tests could be faxed directly from the system. Medications, allergies, past history, family history, social history, and review of systems information could be entered. Medication prescriptions were cross checked for allergies, medication, and disease interactions. Prescriptions could be faxed or printed directly from the system.

SMOS' desire was to become as completely paperless as possible. The AllMeds system contained a messaging e-mail-type application that allowed the practice to avoid the need for notes for prescription refills and other patient calls.

SMOS also wanted the system to assist in improving the flow of patients through the office by tracking where the patient was located in the office, which allowed the physician to know who was ready to be seen and the location of that patient. AllMeds offered all these abilities and was user friendly enough that SMOS could easily shape the system to fit its practice pattern.

SMOS wished to avoid an off-site, Internet-based program, so the practice needed to purchase a local server and firewall. These were configured by the practice's local information technology vendor, which also configured the network and HIPPA-compliant security for the network. Each clinical assistant and physician received a tablet PC. The AllMeds program was also available on all of the existing office PCs. The original interface was with the practice's billing system, which at the time was a UNIX-based system from Medisys.

SMOS described implementation of the EHR as "a retooling of the practice of patient care and documentation." AllMeds Company started training practice staff one month prior to implementation. Prior to this training, an AllMeds representative visited the practice for one day to observe patient flow and to better assess training needs and plan implementation. The formal training session was a two-day event on a Friday and Saturday. The entire staff, at the time, learned all of the basic functionality of the system. Groups were then divided into front office and clinical staff for more intensive training in specific aspects of the EHR program.

The physicians began building stored outlines for rapid entry of history, physical exam, and plans for specific diagnoses. The number of patients to be seen on the date of implementation was not adjusted significantly. This would later be a decision the practice regretted.

On the go-live day, a Wednesday, two AllMeds trainers assisted the practice's staff. Recognizing the practice should have reduced patient numbers by one-half during the go-live period, SMOS did reduce the patient load for the following two weeks.

Implementation was not without challenges, including interruption in the wireless network resulting from proximate location of other wireless networks in the medical office building, and lack of a process for documenting a callback that was in progress or how the call was addressed. Implementation of the EHR at the satellite office in Ft. Payne, Alabama, which subsequently closed for reasons unrelated to the EHR, was delayed pending resolution of challenges and increased comfort in using the EHR.

Six weeks after go-live date, the practice was back to handling its usual number of patients and the staff was leaving the office on time. Staff felt proficient with the system at this point and knew the practice could never go back to the paper-chart system.

SMOS used every aspect of the EHR system. Messages were all handled within the system. All outside paper correspondence was scanned into the patient chart. The practice required absolutely no transcription services. In April 2004, SMOS added computerized x-ray to its capabilities.

In late November 2004, SMOS began serving as a test site for an AllMeds computer scan sheet that covered information including past, family, and social histories, and review of systems form. Use of the sheet saved the practice's clinical assistants a total of two hours per day. In April 2005, a different satellite office was opened in the Birmingham area one day a week. Existing laptops transported to the satellite office were used.

VALUE

Through full use of the EHR, SMOS became more organized and efficient. There were no lost charts. Physicians could review patient records from home. All patient documentation and charges were done on the same date of the patient visit. Physicians did not need to take charts home for later transcription.

Improved efficiency was noted in many areas. Physicians no longer had to wait for the assistants to come out of a patient's room to obtain a history regarding the next patient to be seen. Several employees could be working in the same chart simultaneously. Prescriptions were documented in the EHR clearly and refills were easier to process.

The physicians were able to spend more quality time with the patient. The physician had to perform less of the documentation and thus, had more time for patient care.

Billing staff had immediate desktop access to a patient's record to answer questions regarding procedures performed on a particular date of service. All medical record requests were easily handled. Coding was now supported by documentation. There was a decrease in the number of level 4 and 5 new patient visits that previously did not have necessary documentation to support these codes. With the ease of reporting to referring physicians, consults of level 2 and 3 replaced office visits of lesser codes. Additionally, the practice had been under coding on follow-up patients consistently. Practice revenue from office visits increased.

Transcription cost savings amounted to about $50,000 per year, and with personnel savings, amounted to approximately $75,000 per year. The total cost of SMOS' initial investment in a server, five tablet computers, firewalls, wireless transmitters, network installation, and EHR program and training was $100,000. After the first year, the practice paid approximately $1,000 per month for maintenance, support, and updates.

SMOS' initial research indicated the EHR would pay for itself within 30 months. With the growth of the practice, the calculations indicate the EHR was likely to be at a financial breakeven point after only 20 months.

LESSONS LEARNED

The success of the implementation of EHR at Sports Medicine & Orthopedic Specialists was due to total physician commitment and a dedicated office staff. The practice's leaders indicated both of these qualities are absolutely necessary for any practice to be successful with computerized records. Other lessons learned included:

- Use an IT company that is familiar with network configuration and healthcare.
- Remember an EHR vendor is usually just a software vendor. The integration of the medical record product with the billing system is imperative. A few vendors have products that will function as both systems. In SMOS' research, these products are not as complete in either function.
- The physicians and administrators of a practice must work together to purchase and plan for implementation of the new system. Changes in the work flow and employee responsibilities must be considered before implementation.
- Part of the due-diligence process includes a site visit to one or more practices that are using the computer program. One or more physicians and administrators must take the time to learn the issues that can only come from a site visit.
- Don't ignore the advice received from other practices using the system.

SMOS' leaders conclude with this cautionary advice: "The recommendation to all who are considering EHR is that it will not get any easier to implement this technology in the near future. Government mandates will require the technology within the next 10 years or less. For a new practice, computerized records are an easy beginning. For an established practice, the longer you wait to implement EHR, the more difficult the process."

2005 DAVIES PRIMARY CARE AWARD WINNER
WAYNE OBSTETRICS AND GYNECOLOGY

ABOUT THE PRACTICE

Wayne Obstetrics and Gynecology is a solo physician practice established in 2003 by Jeffrey L. Harris, MD, and located in Jesup, a small town of approximately 10,000 in Southeastern Georgia. Certified in both family practice and obstetrics/gynecology (OB/GYN), Dr. Harris devotes more than 90 percent of his practice to OB/GYN and has a staff of nine, including four FTE nurses, and five administrative/office manager FTEs.

In 2004, the practice had nearly 2,300 patients and 6,000 direct patient encounters. At the time of its Davies Award application, approximately 32 percent of the practice's patients were covered by Medicaid, 14 percent by Blue Cross and Blue Shield, 11 percent by Medicare, and the remainder by numerous other insurance companies.

MANAGEMENT

Harris decided to implement an EHR system prior to opening the practice, and he and the executive office manager selected EncounterPRO® by JMJ Technologies of Atlanta following review of five products from different vendors. They defined specific goals and expectations for the EHR system, including the following:

- Enhance the quality of the patient care visit. Goal: Decrease requests to switch physicians to less than one patient per month.
- Improve accuracy and thoroughness of documentation. Goal: Appropriately increase CPT coding level by 10 percent.
- Decrease exposure to medical liability. Goals: Institute a fax transmittal system of prenatal information flow sheets between the office and hospital, and no malpractice claims filed against the practice.
- Decrease lost productivity and eliminate paper records. Goals: Stop using paper records within six months of implementing the electronic medical record system, and eliminate the need to complete charts after work and on the weekend.
- Improve process efficiency. Goal: Increase patient visits by 10 percent within two years of implementation by increasing available appointments without increasing the number of hours worked.
- Reduce costs and increase profits. Goal: Avoid the normal costs associated with using paper medical records, including supplies for paper charts, employee hours for chart pulls and re-filing, transcription costs, and chart storage space.

Harris, the executive office manager, and assistant office manager coordinated system implementation. The assistant office manager and the registered nurse (RN) were responsible for training. Wayne Obstetrics and Gynecology served as a beta test site for JMJ Technologies.

FUNCTIONALITY AND IMPLEMENTATION

EncounterPRO® data sets included problem lists, procedures, review of systems, medical and nursing diagnosis, medication lists, allergies, demographics, diagnostic test results, radiology results, health maintenance alerts, and E&M coding. The clinical and patient narratives could be captured by free text, template-based text, dictation, or voice recognition.

The EHR's results management capabilities included management of laboratory, radiology, and referral reports. It also kept track of tests for which no results had come back, and generated reports of tests still open, reported overdue tasks, and assigned responsibility for overdue items.

The CPOE system encompassed electronic prescription writing, lab orders, x-ray orders, nursing entries (vitals screen), and referrals. All orders were highly configurable and could be part of the work flow.

The EHR had an internal messaging system that allowed for increased communication among members of the healthcare team. It created to-do items for the providers that were attached to both the history of the to-do item and the patient's chart. Messages were routed through work flow or by selecting specific recipients.

To provide patient support, the EHR offered a patient take-home report that included all care instructions, a summary of all labs or tests ordered by the physician, and a list of all medications and instructions.

The EHR was integrated with a billing/scheduling system that supplied information about appointments, schedules and patient demographics. It also had a third-party interface showing the front office staff which specialists and labs were covered by which insurance companies.

Structured data permitted queries against open and closed assessments, drug history, family history, and other elements.

EncounterPRO was a client/server application that ran on Microsoft Windows® 2000 Server and Microsoft SQL Server™ 2000. The EHR fully interfaced with more than 20 practice management systems, and a laboratory interface was also available from the vendor.

The technology had very few issues that required management. As a new practice, Wayne Obstetrics and Gynecology purchased its server and all other hardware through JMJ Technologies. The practice chose to blend a combination of flat touch screen Wyse solid state terminals in the front office and exam rooms with Acer tablet PCs for the physician and nurses.

The practice's first step was to implement the practice management system and become familiar with its use, which occurred in August 2003. By October 2003 the practice was ready to implement the EMR. EncounterPro training was performed onsite for one week during which the practice went live with the system by the third day. All documentation has been performed in EncounterPro ever since, with all use of paper records stopped within three months.

VALUE

The practice successfully achieved the business objectives of EHR implementation, as outlined earlier. In meeting the objective of enhanced quality of the patient care visit, since implementation of the EHR, patient requests to transfer records (other than patients moving out of the area) were consistently less than one per month.

In meeting the objective of improved accuracy and thoroughness of documentation, the most significant finding was an increase in coding from level 2 to level 3 visits of nearly 17 percent for established patients and an eight percent increase in level 4 visits for new patients.

In meeting the objective of decreased exposure to medical liability, no liability suits had occurred at the time of its Davies Award application since implementation of the EHR system.

In meeting the goals associated with increased productivity and eliminating paper records, paper records were discontinued three months after implementation of the EMR system, well ahead of the goal of six months. The number of work hours to document patient encounters by the provider decreased by an average of four hours per week while simultaneously increasing the number of patients that were seen by 225 percent.

In meeting the objective of improved process efficiency, patient visits increased from an average of 311 patients per month in 2003 to 500 patients per month in 2004 to 735 patients per month in 2005. Two additional FTEs were added to meet the increased clinical demands of more patient visits. No additional members were required to maintain the EHR due to the increased productivity.

In meeting the goal associated with reducing costs and increasing profits, the practice avoided the cost of square footage for a records room, as this was not needed. At least one FTE of clerical support was not hired because there was no need to maintain paper records and filing.

LESSONS LEARNED

Wayne Obstetrics and Gynecology cited many lessons learned, including the importance of being patient and properly "doing your homework" to research EHR products, and that training was almost as important as what product the practice selected in the first place. "The training with EncounterPro was outstanding. Make sure you understand how your staff will be trained (onsite or Web-based), how much training you will receive, and who will help when you have questions after the training is over."

On the topic of start up, which for this practice included purchasing hardware, practice management software, and EHR software, ensure everyone understands their respective roles in the setup process to avoid any confusion or delays.

In the design of office space, understand what the practice wishes to accomplish with its EHR system. As a new practice, Wayne Obstetrics and Gynecology chose a hybrid model of fixed terminals and portable tablet PCs, which worked well for the practice. Plan adequate space for a dedicated server room that is secured, properly cooled, and dust free (not a converted closet).

In summary, the practice indicated the following: "EncounterPro works in synergy with the physician and staff to meet the most important goal of all, the highest quality of medical care for all the patients of Wayne Obstetrics and Gynecology."

Index

A

Access control, 99, 100
Accountability, 99
ACUMEN, 45, 46, 47
Acute care, operational data for, 73
Admission, discharge, and transfer (ADT) data, 57
Advanced Clinical Information System (ACIS), 71–75
Advanced patient tracking, 36
Adverse drug reaction monitoring system, 52
Adverse events
    detection of, 36
    prevention of, 31
Advice rules, 40
    programming for, 41
Age-related alerts, 123
Agfa-Bayer PACS system, 91, 94, 111
A⁴ Health Systems'® HealthMatics EMR Electronic Medical Record, 148
Alert fatigue, 66
Alerts
    age-related, 123
    allergy, 123, 160
    alternative drug, 43
    best-practice, 43
    practice, 66
Allergy alerts, 123, 160
AllMeds Company, 167–170
Alpha SQL Server, 94
Alternative drug alerts, 43
Ambulatory patient record system (COSTAR), 77
Analog data, management of, 29
Ancillary interface for the CIS, 69
Ancillary services, interface of, via HL7, 68, 69
ANSI-M technology, 79
Application training, 99
Automated charge capture functionality, 144
Automated medical record system (AMRS), 77, 78
    limitations to, 77
Automated patient records, planning for, 39–40
Automatic data processing application coordinator, 24
Automatic discharge summaries, 36
Automatic prompts for communication, 36

B

Babbitt, Nancy R., 143, 145
Baldridge Award, 1
Baptist Sports Medicine and Orthopedics Specialists, 167
Bar Code Medication Administration and VISTA Imaging, 84
Baselet fragments, 69
Baselets, 69
Bat, Thomas E., 147, 148
Bess Kaiser Hospital, 57
Best-of-breed approach, 6–7, 102, 104
Best-practice alerts, 43
Best practices, 43, 123
"Big bang" approach, 98, 113
Billing improvements, 12, 13
Blue Cross of Georgia, 139
Boards of directors, leadership role of, 3
Brigham and Women's Hospital (Boston), 31–38
    challenges created by organizational evolution, 34–35
    changing technology and functionality, 35–36
    clinical information system at, 15
    electronic health record's effect on healthcare in, 36–37
    functionality, 32–33
    lessons to share, 37–38
    management, 31–32
    technology, 33
    value, 33–34
Brigham Integrated Computing System (BICS), 31–38
    development and implementation, 31–32
    functional objectives of, 32–33
    measurement and analysis of, 33–34
    technological development of, 33
Browser-technology-based systems, 115
Business case, establishing, for electronic health record implementation, 4–5

C

Cabletron Hub-based network, at North Mississippi Health Services, 50, 51
CARE, 54, 55
Care continuum, patient movement through, 12
Carrot-and-stick approach, 6
Caseload management, 88
Center for Information Technology Leadership, 37
Cerner Corporation, 97
Change control planning, 91
Charges, capturing, 13
Chart audits, 140–141
Charting, 68
    electronic, 9, 115
    flow, 87
    intravenous, 115
    online medication, 9
Chart review, 62–63, 68
Chief executive officer (CEO), leadership by, 2–3, 6

Children's Hospital Boston, 37
Cincinnati Children's Hospital Medical Center, 115–119
    boards of directors leadership at, 3
    communications at, 10
    electronic health record planning committees at, 3
    functionality, 117
    management of, 115–117
    medication error decline at, 9
    patient safety and, 8
    regulatory compliance at, 11
    risk management at, 6
    technology, 118
    training program at, 7
    user acceptance as risk factor at, 5
    value, 118–119
Cincinnati Children's Hospital Research Foundation, 115
Citizens Memorial Healthcare (Missouri), 127–131
    automatic charge capture at, 14
    CEO leadership at, 3
    change resistance as risk factor at, 5
    communications at, 10
    electronic records at, 9
    functionality, 129
    IS Steering Committee at, 3–4
    management of, 127–128
    net patient revenues at, 12
    order entry at, 10
    patient safety and, 8
    positive return at, 4
    risk assessment at, 5
    technology, 130
    value, 130–131
Citrix Secure Gateway, 130
Citrix WinFrame, 74
Clinical command center, creation of, 102
Clinical Content Consultants, LLC, 140
Clinical data, integrity of, 21, 29
Clinical decision support system
    at Group Health Cooperative of Puget Sound, 43
    at North Mississippi Health Services, 51
    at Riverpoint Pediatrics, 160
    at Roswell Pediatric Center, 144
Clinical documentation, 115
Clinical Information at Queen's (CLiQ), 71–75
    clinician satisfaction with, 73
    data entry in, 73
    implementation of, 72
    Quick Scan, 73
Clinical information systems (CISs)
    at Brigham and Women's Hospital, 15, 31
    at Columbia-Presbyterian Medical Center, 19, 20, 21–22
    at Intermountain Healthcare, 27

at Kaiser Permanente Colorado Region, 67–70
at Kaiser Permanente Northwest, 57
at Kaiser Permanente of Ohio, 45
at Northwestern Memorial Hospital, 61
at Queen's Medical Center, 71–75
Clinically Related Information System (CRIS) project at Group Health Cooperative of Puget Sound, 39–44
functionality of, 40
goals of, 39–40
implementation of, 41
Clinical performance improvement, 74–75
Clinical research, computer-based patient record system in facilitating, 64
Clinician's Desktop, 87
CMT Interface as external interface for the CIS, 69
Coded data entry, 69
Colorado Permanente Medical Group (CPMG), 67
Columbia-Presbyterian Medical Center (New York City), 14, 19–22
clinical information system at, 19, 20, 21–22
Event Monitor program at, 20
functionality, 20
integrated advanced information management system at, 19
management of, 19
Medical Entities Dictionary at, 19
technology, 20–21
value, 21–22
Common user interface, 9
Communications
in addressing implementation risks, 5
automatic prompts for, 36
digital imaging and, 55
functionality of, 110
increased, 10
nurse-to-nurse, 117
physician-patient, 66
Community-based services, 85, 125
Compliance with pain assessment, 11
Computer-based Patient Record Institute (CPRI), 1
Computer-based patient records, 61, 77
Computer-based systems, implementation of, 1
Computerized clinical order entry (COE), 115
Computerized patient record system (CPRS), 81
automated practitioner order entry into, 82
decision support features, 83
functionality of, 82–83
implementation of, 82
training for, 82
Computerized practitioner order entry (CPOE)
at Brigham and Women's Hospital, 32
at Citizens Memorial Healthcare, 127, 128, 129
at Cooper Pediatrics, 136
at Evanston Northwestern Healthcare, 121
at Wayne Obstetrics and Gynecology, 172

Confidentiality
    data integrity and, 60
    training and, 99–100
Consistency of care, improving, 9
Continuous quality improvement, 64
Continuum of care, 6, 124, 153
Controlled medical terminology (CMT), 68, 69
Cooper, Jeffrey D., 135
Cooper Pediatrics (Georgia), 135–137
    functionality and implementation, 135–136
    lessons learned, 137
    management, 135
    value, 136–137
Costs, minimizing, 95
Cranshaw, Janet, 155
Cross-departmental teams, 128
Cross-functional teams, 4, 86
Crystal Reports and Business Objects, 105
Custom formularies, 69
Customized decision support tools, 144

D

Data. *See also* Information
    admission, discharge, and transfer, 57
    components of, 93
    encoded, 29
    encounter, 140
    integrity of clinical, 21, 29
    management of analog, 29
    operational for acute care, 73
    structured, 172
Database
    MicroMedex drug, 73
    MUMPS, 94
    structured query language (SQL) server-based, 41
Database backups, 21
Data capture tools, 122
Data dictionary, 94
Data entry
    coded, 69
    duplication of, 110
    keyboard, 58, 111
    reducing errors in, 51–52
    three-screen approach to, 144
Data exchange
    Health Level Seven (HL7) protocol for, 20
    standards in, 55
Data integrity, 55
    confidentiality and, 60
    security and, 84, 98
DataTree MUMPS, 33
Davies, Nicholas E., 1

Davies, Nicholas E., Award Program, 1–2

Davies Framework for Evaluating Electronic Health Records, 2

Decentralized Hospital Computer Program (DHCP), 14, 23, 26

    expansion of clinical functionality of, 24–25

    track record for extensibility, 26

Decision support

    at Cincinnati Children's Hospital Medical Center, 117

    at Evanston Northwestern Healthcare, 123

    at Group Health Cooperative of Puget Sound, 43

    at Harvard Vanguard Medical Associates, 79

    at Heritage Behavioral Health Center, Inc., 87–88

    at Kaiser Permanente Northwest, 59

    at Maimonides Medical Center, 8

    Medical Automated Record System as, at Kaiser Permanente of Ohio, 46

    at Ohio State University Health System, 93

    at Queens Health Network, 3, 110

    in reducing medication errors, 8

    at Regenstrief Institute for Health Care, 54

    at Riverpoint Pediatrics, 160

    at Roswell Pediatric Center, 144

Define, Measure, Analyze, Improve, and Control (DMAIC) process improvement approach, 7, 115

Digital imaging and communications in medicine (DICOM), 55

Disease management, 64, 140

Docs Inc. (Fayetteville, Arkansas), 155

Document imaging, 99

Downtime

    planning for, 130

    as risk factor, 5

Drop-down pick lists, 58

Drug interactions, 63

Due-diligence process, 170

E

Eclipsys 7000, 71, 73

Education in addressing implementation risks, 5

80/20 Rule, 65

Electronic charting and discharge, 9

Electronic clinical records, 115

Electronic data sets, using consistent, 9

Electronic discharge instructions, 11

Electronic health records (EHRs). *See also* Medical records; Patient records

    at Brigham and Women's Hospital, 37

    at Citizens Memorial Healthcare, 127–131

    at Citizens Memorial Healthcare (Missouri), 9

    at Cooper Pediatrics, 135–137

    at Evans Medical Group, 139–141

    at Evanston Northwestern Healthcare, 121–125

    at Group Health Cooperative of Puget Sound 40, (Washington), 42–43

    at Harvard Vanguard Medical Associates, 77–80

    at Heritage Behavioral Health Center, Inc., 85–89

    at Intermountain Health Care, 14–15, 28–29

    at Maimonides Medical Center, 101–107

MedicaLogic, 74
   at North Fulton Family Medicine, 147–150
   at North Mississippi Health Services, 49–52
   at Northwestern Memorial Hospital, 61–64
   at Ohio State University Health System, 9–10, 91 95
   at Old Harding Pediatrics Associates, 151–153
   at Pediatrics at the Basin, 155–157
   planning for, 3
   at Queen Health Network, 109–114
   at Riverpoint Pediatrics, 159–161
   at Roswell Pediatric Center, 143–145
   at Southeast Texas Medical Associates, LLP, 163–165
   at Sports Medicine & Orthopedic Specialists, PC, 167–170
   successful implementation of, 1
   at Veterans Affairs, U.S. Department of, 23, 24
   VistA, 14
   at Wayne Obstetrics and Gynecology, 171–174
Electronic medication charting, 115
Electronic practice management (EPM) systems at Southeast Texas Medical Associates, LLP, 163
Electronic signatures, 9
E-LINK, 124
Elmhurst Hospital Center (Queens, New York), 109
Encoded data, 29
Encounter data, 140
EncounterPRO®
   at Cooper Pediatrics, 135, 136
   at Riverpoint Pediatrics, 159, 160
   at Wayne Obstetrics and Gynecology, 171–174
Encounter System, 45
End-to-end process redesign, 124
End-to-end system integration, 124
End-user support planning, 91
Enterprise Data Warehouse (EDW), 72
EpicCare®. *See also* Epic Systems
   at Group Health Cooperative of Puget Sound, 42–43
   at Harvard Vanguard Medical Associates, 77, 78, 79
   at Kaiser Permanente Northwest, 57–60
   at Northwestern Memorial Hospital, 62
Epic Systems. *See also* EpicCare®
   at Evanston Northwestern Healthcare, 121–125
   at Group Health Cooperative of Puget Sound, 42–43
   at Harvard Vanguard Medical Associates, 78
   at Kaiser Permenente Northwest, 59
Evaluation & management (E&M) coding, 135–136
Evans (Georgia) Medical Group, 139–141
   functionality and implementation, 140
   lessons learned, 141
   management, 139
   value, 140–141
Evanston (Illinois)Healthcare
   change in medication procedures at, 9
   staff-related reductions at, 12

Evanston (Illinois)Hospital, 121
Evanston (Illinois) Northwestern Healthcare, 121–125
    building of financial case for, 4
    capturing of charges at, 13
    electronic health record planning committees at, 3
    functionality, 122–123
    goals at, 3
    leadership at, 3
    management, 121–122
    Medical Informatics department at, 3
    patient safety and, 8
    technology, 123–124
    value, 124–125
Evidence-based guidelines, 9

F

Feinberg School of Medicine, 121
Field defaults, 58
Flow charting, 87
4 Roles of Leadership® model, 128
FranklinCovey's The 4 Roles of Leadership® model, 128
Free text reports, 29

G

GE Centricity, 136
Gemini Executive Implementation Committee, 97
Gemini Project, 97–100
    functionality of, 98–99
    primary objective of, 98–99
    value of, 100
Glaser, John, 15
Glenbrook (Illinois)Hospital, 121
Godstein, Denise, 167
Goldstein, Samuel, 167
Gonzalzles, Armand A., 159
Graphical user interface (GUI), 69
Group Health Cooperative of Puget Sound (Washington), 39–44
    clinical decision support, 43
    EHR system and implementation, 42–43
    functionality, 40
    lessons learned, 43–44
    management, 39–40
    objectives of new EHR system, 42
    technology, 40–41
    value, 41–42, 43
GUI as external interface for the CIS, 69

H

Harding Behavioral Health Hospital (Columbus, Ohio), 91
Hard return on investment (ROI), 7, 12
Harris, Jeffrey L., 171
Harvard Community Health Plan, 77

Harvard Pilgrim Health Care, 77

Harvard's Countway Library of Medicine, 37

Harvard Vanguard Medical Associates (Boston), 77–80

    functionality, 77–79

    management, 77–78

    technology, 79–80

    value, 80

Healthcare

    effectiveness of, 110

    efficiency of, 110

    improving patient safety in, 8

Healthcare Information and Management Systems Society (HIMSS), 1

    Davies, Nicholas E., Award Program, 1–2

Healthcare information technology, clinical benefits of, 6

Health Evaluation through Logical Processing (HELP), 14, 27–30

    data collection requirements of, 28

Health Insurance Portability and Accountability Act (HIPAA) (1996), 11, 103, 130

Health Level Seven (HL7) protocol

    at Citizens Memorial Healthcare, 130

    at Columbia-Presbyterian Medical Center, 20

    at Harvard Vanguard Medical Associates, 80

    at Kaiser Permanente Colorado Region, 68, 69

    at Pediatrics at the Basin, 155

    at Veterans Affairs Puget Sound Healthcare System, 84

Health maintenance rules, 63

HealthMatics Ntierprise Practice Management System (North Fulton, Georgia), 148

Health Network Architecture (HNA) Millennium, 97

Health Plan Employer Plan Data and Information Set (HEDIS), 80, 149

Healthwise® Knowledgebase, 43

Heritage Behavioral Health Center, Inc. (Decatur, Illinois), 85–89

    concern over lost productivity and staff resistance at, 5

    cost savings at, 13

    cross-functional teams at, 4

    functionality, 87–88

    management, 85–86

    revenue increase at, 13–14

    technology, 88

    training and certification program at, 5

    value, 88–89

Heritage Network (Decatur, Illinois), 85, 86

    development of, 85–86

Hickham, John B., 53

Highland Park (Illinois) Hospital, 121

Holistic planning process, 6

Homegrown systems, 37

HSIS (Echo Group), 87

I

IBM High Availability Cluster Multi-Processing (HACMP) software, 123

ICD-9 codes, 11

ID passwords, 123

IHCNet, 15

Illinois, University of (at Chicago) Medical Center, 97–100
    business case at, 4–5
    functionality, 98–99
    management, 97–98
    reallocation of nurse time, 13
    technology, 99–100
    value, 100
    vendor selection and, 4
Implementation planning, 6–7, 91, 122
Indiana University Hospitals, 139
Information. *See also* Data
    access to referring physician, 9
    maximizing access to, 95
    point-of-care availability of real-time patient, 8–9
    timeliness of, 110
    as tool in quality improvement programs, 36
Information warehouse, 93
InfoScriber (Conundrum Inc.), 87
Infrastructure and hardware preparation planning, 91
Input message editing, 51
Integrated advanced information management system (IAMS), 19
Integrated systems strategy, 6
Integrating Clinical Informatics System (ICIS), 115–119
    implementation of, 116–117
Intermountain Health Care (IHC) (Salt Lake City), 7, 27–30
    electronic health record installation at, 14–15
    functionality, 28–29
    Health Evaluation through Logical Processing (HELP), 14, 27–30
    Informatics Council of, 28
    management, 27–28
    technology, 29–30
    value, 30
InterSystems Cache, 33
Intravenous charting, 115
INVISION system, 116

J

James, Arthur G., Cancer Hospital (Columbus, Ohio), 91
Jericho Project, 87
JMJ Technologies (Atlanta), 159, 171–172
Joint Commission on Accreditation of Healthcare Organizations (JCAHO)
    patient safety and, 8, 124
    security and confidentiality requirements, 103
    standards for restraint orders, 74
Just-in-time training, 7, 102, 116

K

Kaiser Foundation Health Plan, 67
Kaiser Permanente Colorado region, 67–68
    functionality, 68–69
    management, 67
    technology, 69–70

value, 70
Kaiser Permanente Northwest (Washington), 57–60
    functionality, 58–59
    management, 57–58
    technology, 59–60
    value, 60
Kaiser Permanente of Ohio, 45–52
    functionality, 46–47
    management, 45–46
    technology, 47
    value, 48
Kaiser Sunnyside Medical Center (Salem, Oregon), 57
Keyboard entry, 58, 111
Khoury, Allan, 45
KnowledgeLinks, 36

L

Lamberts, Robert, 139, 141
Leadership
    by boards of directors, 3
    by chief executive officers, 2–3, 6
    by medical directors, 3
    project risk and, 5
    vendor selection and, 4
Lifetime electronic clinical records, 115
Logician, 139, 140
Longitudinal medical record (LMR), 35
Lost productivity as risk factor, 5
Loveys, Alice, 155
"Lowest-hanging fruit" principle, 53–54
Lytec, 160

M

Maimonides Access Clinical System (MACS), 101–107
    embedding evidence-based care and consensus-based practice guidelines in, 105
    implementation of, 106
Maimonides Medical Center (Brooklyn, New York), 101–107
    challenges at, 104–105
    communications at, 10
    decision support system at, 8
    decline in auxiliary tests, 9
    drop in problem medication orders at, 8
    effect on care, 105–106
    functionality, 103
    implementation of PACs and voice recognition systems at, 13
    improved bill collection at, 14
    just-in-time training at, 7
    leadership of, 2–3
    lessons learned, 106–107
    management of, 101–102
    medication delivery at, 10
    patient visits to emergency room at, 12

regulatory compliance at, 11
technology, 103–104
value, 104
vendor selection and, 4
Massachusetts General Hospital (MGH), 34
Utility Multi-Programming System, 25
Materials and staffing reductions, 12
McDonald, Clement J., 53, 139
McKay-Dee Medical Center (Ogden, Utah), 28
Medical Automated Record System (MARS), 45–52
Medical directors, leadership of, 3
Medical Entities Dictionary (MED), 19
Medical Logic Modules (MLMs), 20
MedicaLogic, 139
Encounter Form Editor program, 139
Medical records. *See also* Electronic health records (EHRS); patient records
automated, 77
employee shifting and, 12
longitudinal, 35
Regenstrief system of, 53, 139
universal format for, 87
Medication orders, pharmacist interventions in, 8
Medications
allergy alerts and, 123
decline in transcription errors with online charting, 9
delivery of, 10
electronic charting of, 115
evaluation of orders for drug interactions, 30
management support, 87, 88
reducing errors in, 8
Medispan® drug database, 148
MEDITECH system, 128, 129, 130
Med/IV charting platform, 117
MEDPATH, 20
MedSTAR, 45
Mental health services, 85
Metrics, 11–12
Meyer, Greg, 155
MicroMedex drug database, 73
Miner, Cherie, 167
Morrow, James R., 147, 148, 149
Mount Sinai School of Medicine, 101, 109
MS Word 97, 87
Multimedia computer-based interactive training, 58
Multi-step algorithms, 36
MUMPS database, 33, 94
DataTree, 33

N

National Council for Prescription Drug Programs (NCPDP), 55
National Library of Medicine, 61, 65
funding of integrated advanced information system by, 19

Needs assessment, 91

NetReach project at Northwestern Memorial Hospital, 61, 64, 65

Network integration, 20

New York City Health and Hospitals Corporation, 109

NextGen™ Healthcare Information Services, 163

North Fulton Family Medicine (Georgia), 147–150

    functionality and implementation, 148–149

    lessons learned, 149–150

    management, 147

    value, 149

North Mississippi Health Services (Tupelo), 49–52

    functionality, 50–51

    management of, 49–50

    technology, 51–52

    value, 52

North Mississippi Medical Center (Tupelo), 49

Northwestern Memorial Corporation, 61

Northwestern Memorial Hospital (Evanston), 61–64

    challenges addressed, 65

    functionality, 62–63

    lessons to be shared, 65–66

    management, 61–62

    technology, 63

    value, 63–64

Northwestern University's Feinberg School of Medicine, 121

Nurse-to-nurse communication orders, 117

O

Ohio State University Health System, 91–95

    cash flow improvements at, 14

    cross-functional teams at, 4

    electronic health records at, 9–10

    functionality, 92–93

    implementation of PACs at, 13

    IT team leadership at, 4

    length of inpatient stays at, 12

    management, 91–92

    medication delivery at, 10

    patient safety and, 8

    regulatory compliance at, 11

    technology, 93–94

    value, 94–95

Ohio State University Hospitals, 91

Old Harding Pediatric Associates (Tennessee), 151–153

    functionality and implementation, 152–153

    lessons learned, 153

    management, 151

    value, 153

Online medication charting, decline in transcription errors, 9

OPENLink™, 118

Operational data for acute care, 73

Operational planning, 91

Order entry, 63

P

Pareto's Principle, 65

Partners Healthcare System hospitals, 34–35

Passavant Hospital, 61

Passwords, 11

Patient(s)

    advanced tracking of, 36

    audit trial showing access to data of, 21

    check-in of, 9

    protecting confidentiality of, 58

    satisfaction of, 64

    support for, 136

    throughput of, 106

    timeliness of information of, 110

Patient capacity management, 106

Patient Care and Access Process Initiatives (PCAPI), 116

Patient care encounter, 25

Patient data exchange, 25

Patient flow, 12

Patient Gateway, 36

Patient records. *See also* Electronic health records (EHRs); Medical records

    ambulatory, 77

    availability and completeness of, 64

    computer-based, 61, 77, 81–84

Patient safety, 7

    efforts to improve, 8–10

    targeted dimensions of, 110

Patient SnapShot, 63

Pediatrics at the Basin (Pittsford, New York), 155–157

    functionality and implementation, 155–156

    lessons learned, 157

    management, 155

    value, 156–157

Per-Se Technologies, 111

Physician information, access to referring, 9

Physician order entry, 113

Physician-patient communication, 66

Physician practice style, 152, 153

Physicians Advisory Group, leadership role of, 3

Physicians' Current Procedural Terminology (CPT®) codes, 167–168

Picture archiving and communication system (PACS), 36

    implementation of, 13

Planning teams, composition of, 6

Point-and-click procedure

    at Kaiser Permanente Colorado Region, 68

    at North Fulton Family Medicine, 148

    at Roswell Pediatric Center, 144

Point-of-care availability of real-time patient information, 8–9

Point-of-care capability, 124

Point-to-text encoding system, 29

Practice alerts, 66

Process improvements, 7, 11–12

Process re-engineering, 107, 112

Productivity, lost, as risk factor, 5

Project governance, 7

Project Infocare, 127–131, 130

    implementation of, 128, 130–131

Project Jericho, 85

    business expectations, 88–89

Project risk, leadership and, 5

Protocol for electronic mail transfer, transmission control protocol/Internet protocol (TCP/IP) as, 26

Q

Quality improvement, continuous, 64

Quality improvement checklist (QUIC) application, Veterans Health Administration use of, 26

Quality improvement programs, information technology as tool in, 36

Quality of care

    improvements in, 137

    indicators of, 41

    targeted dimensions of, 110

Quantifiable returns, 11–12

Queen's Clinical Performance Improvement model, 71–72

Queens Health Network (New York), 100–114

    current status and lessons to share, 112–114

    functionality, 110–111

    increased communications at, 10

    leadership at, 3

    management, 100–110

    PACs and voice recognition systems at, 13

    pharmacist interventions in medication orders, 8

    regulatory compliance at, 11

    revenue increase at, 13

    technology, 111

    value, 112

Queen's Health System (Oahu), 71

Queens Hospital Center (QHC), 109

Queen's Medical Center (QMC) (Hawaii), 71–75

    functionality, 72–73

    management, 71–72

    technology, 73–74

    value, 74–75

R

Radiology, reallocation of resources in, 12

Real-time patient information, point-of-care availability of, 8–9

Regenstrief, Samuel N., 53

Regenstrief Institute for Health Care (Indianapolis), 7, 53–56

    functionality, 53–55

    management, 53

    technology, 55

    value, 55–56

Regenstrief Medical Records System (RMRS), 139

primary goal of, 53

Regulatory compliance, 7

Relational database management system (RDBMS), 69

Remote access, 123, 130

Resource shifting, 12

Results reporting system (RRS), 57

Return on investment (ROI), 2, 7–14

    hard, 7, 12

    soft, 7–8

Risk assessments, 4–5, 6

Riverpoint Pediatrics (Illinois), 159–161

    functionality and implementation, 159–160

    lessons learned, 161

    management, 159

    value, 160–161

Rochester Health Commission, 156

Role-based training, 116

Roswell Pediatric Center (Georgia), 143–145

    functionality and implementation, 144

    lessons learned, 145

    management, 143–144

    value, 144–145

Rule-based reminder system, 54, 55

Rules-based logic, application to patient data, 27

Rules engine, 115

S

Secure Sockets Layer (SSL) encryption, 123

Security, data integrity and, 84, 98

Security protocols, 11

Selection lists, 58

Self-service data-reporting tools, 105

Sequoia Software Corporation, 45

Shadow backup, 33

Siemens Medical Solutions Health Services Corporation, 116

Site visits, 2

Six Sigma's Define, Measure, Analyze, Improve, and Control (DMAIC) process improvement approach, 7, 115

SmartRx, 59

SmartSets, 59

SOAP (simple object access protocol) note format

    at North Fulton Family Medicine, 148

    at Old Harding Pediatric Associates, 152–153

    at Sports Medicine & Orthopedic Specialists, PC, 167

SOAPware at Pediatrics at the Basin, 155, 156

Soft return on investment, 7–8

Solove, Richard J., Research Institute, 91

Southeast Texas Medical Associates, LLP (SETMA), 163–165

    functionality and implementation, 163–164

    lessons learned, 165

    management, 163

    value, 164

Sports Medicine & Orthopedic Specialists, PC (Alabama), 167–170
    functionality and implementation, 167–169
    lessons learned, 170
    management, 167
    value, 169
Staff buy-in as risk factor, 5
Staff resistance as risk factor, 5
Strategic planning
    at Citizens Memorial Healthcare, 127
    at Heritage Behavioral Health Center, Inc., 85
    at Old Harding Pediatric Associates, 151
    role of boards of directors in, 3
String-matching, 58
Structured data, 172
Structured project management process, 40–41
Structured query language (SQL) server-based database, 41
Summary lists, Joint Commission on Accreditation of Healthcare Organizations (JCAHO)-mandated, 11
Synonym matching, 58
Systematized Nomenclature of Medicine (SNOMED) codes, 69
System data integrity, 51–52
    monitoring accuracy, completeness and, 21–22
System integration, 114
Systems re-engineering, 87
System templates, 58

T
Tablet PCs, 160
Talk Technologies, 111
Team Jericho, 86
TeleVox Lab Calls, 148
Touch screen monitor systems, 160
Training
    application, 99
    confidentiality and, 99–100
    just-in-time, 7, 102, 116
    multimedia computer-based interactive, 58
    role-based, 116
Transcription, decline in errors in, 9
Transmission control protocol/Internet protocol (TCP/IP), as protocol for electronic mail transfer, 26
Treatment planning support, 87–88
Trickle-down effect, 141
Turnaround time improvements, 118

U
Ulticare/Patient 1 system, 111
Universal access to workstations, 32
Universal record format, 87
User authentication, 99, 100
User-centric approach, 55
User satisfaction, 64, 79
    maximizing, 95
User surveys, 57

V

Vaccine information sheets, 153
Value, 7–14
Vendor selection
 leadership role in, 4
 responsibility, 4
Veterans Affairs, U.S. Department of (VA), 23–26
 FileMan, 25
 functionality, 24–25
 Information Resources Advisory Council (IRAC) at, 24
 management, 23–24
 quality improvement checklist application at, 26
 technology, 25–26
 value, 26
Veterans Affairs medical centers (VAMC), 23, 25
Veterans Affairs Puget Sound Health Care System (Washington), 81–84
 functionality, 82–83
 management, 81–82
 technology, 83–84
 value, 84
Veterans Health Administration (VHA), 14
 Decentralized Hospital Computer Program (DHCP) at, 14, 23, 24–25, 26
Veterans Health Information Systems & Technology (VISTA), 83–74
Viritual storage access method, 47
Virtual memory system (VMS), 25
Virtual private network (VPN), 35
Virtual storage extended/enterprise services architecture (VSE/ESA) operating system, 51
Visit notes at North Fulton Family Medicine, 148
VistA EHR, 14
Voice capture/transcription, 68
Voice over IP (VoIP) phones, 124

W

Wagner, Arnold, Jr., 125
Warfarin toxicity, 9
Warner, Homer R., 27
Wayne Obstetrics and Gynecology (Georgia), 171–174
 functionality and implementation, 172
 lessons learned, 173–174
 management, 171
 value, 173
Wesley Hospitals, 61
Wide-area network, real-time date entry and retrival by, 50
Work flow
 at Cooper Pediatrics, 135, 136
 at Queens Health Network, 110
 at Riverpoint Pediatrics, 159–160
 at Southeast Texas Medical Associates, LLP, 164

Y

Yellow-sticker charging, 130